HOW TO FORTIFY YOUR IMMUNE SYSTEM

HOW TO FORTIFY YOUR IMMUNE SYSTEM

Donald E. Dickenson

PH.D.

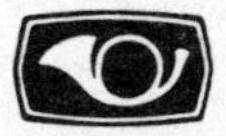

Arlington Books
Clifford Street Mayfair
London

HOW TO FORTIFY
YOUR IMMUNE SYSTEM
First published 1984 by
Arlington Books (Publishers) Ltd
3 Clifford Street, Mayfair
London W1

© 1984 Donald E. Dickenson

Typeset by Preface Ltd, Salisbury
Printed and bound by
Billings & Sons, Worcester

British Library Cataloguing in Publication Data

Dickenson, Donald E.
How to fortify your immune system.
1. Immunology
I. Title
616.07'9   QR181

ISBN 0 85140 633 5

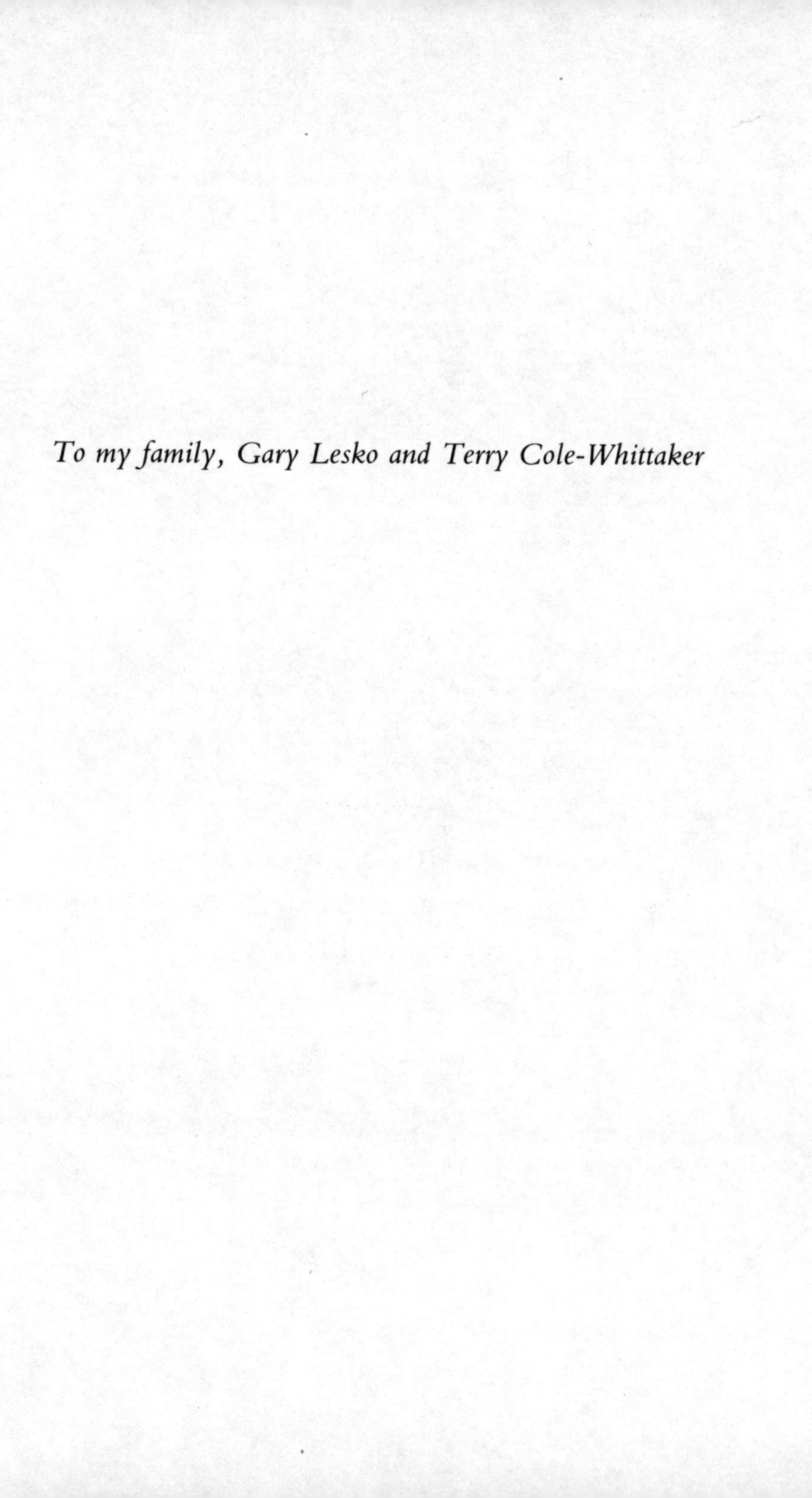

To my family, Gary Lesko and Terry Cole-Whittaker

Acknowledgements

I would like to thank the educators and scientists whose research and writings have contributed to this book.

My special thanks to Dr. Eric Pearl for his support, humor and editorial assistance.

I would like to thank Dr. Garyx Zimmerman, Mrs. Sylvia Fahlman, Mrs. Rae Sincher, Mr. Phillip Marx, Mr. David Goodstein and my patients and friends whose indelible love and support mean more than they know.

My profound thanks to my publisher, Mr. Desmond Elliott, whose patience, courage and commitment have made this book possible.

Contents

Introduction

This book is written in three parts. The first part refers to the relationship between disease and immunity and nutrition. The second and more technical part is an explanation of the different 'soldiers' of the immune system and is necessary for a more complete understanding of the immune system. From the second part one gains an appreciation for the diversity and efficiency of the human immune system. The third part comprises the 'list of ingredients' required to fortify the immune system and connects each nutrient to an immune system function or dysfunction.

A glossary is provided at the beginning to assist the reader in understanding the technical terms and a fuller appreciation of the book will be gained if this is studied first. The numbers in the body of the text identify the references.

This book is intended for information purposes only and is designed to be an adjunct to professional guidance. The author stresses the concept of personal individuality and neither he nor the publisher can be responsible for the inappropriate usage of the information contained herein.

Glossary

Ascorbic acid: Vitamin C. The vitamin which provides for wound healing, resistance to infections and maintains capillary integrity as an essential for proline hydroxylation in collagen synthesis; enhances iron absorption and facilitates conversion of folic to folinic acid.

Adrenal gland: An endocrine gland located on top of each kidney responsible for producing adrenalin, corticosteroids and other hormones.

Alternative pathway of complement activation: One of the two pathways of activating the complement system not requiring the presence of antibodies.

Amine: A substance containing carbon atoms and ammonia and having hormone-like activity.

Amino acids: The basic building units of proteins.

Amyl Nitrite: A volatile inflammable organic liquid used in the treatment of suffocation resulting from attacks of angina pectoris. When sharp spells of this distressing ailment come on, the inhalation of Amyl Nitrite usually gives relief. This chemical is also used as a 'recreational' drug.

Antibody: Y-shaped proteins capable of neutralizing

foreign invading organisms and some tumor cells. An antibody is produced as a result of introducing an antigen and is capable of specifically combining with the antigen.

Antigen: A substance that can cause a detectable immune response.

Antigen-antibody complex: A complex formed when an antibody combines with an antigen.

Antimicrobial: Having the capacity to neutralize a microscopic organism such as a disease-producing bacterium.

Antioxidant: A substance which protects the body from the destructive properties of oxygen or peroxide. This process aids in retarding aging.

Arginine (L-Arginine): A basic, six-carbon amino acid found in proteins.

Atrophy: To waste away, wither.

Autoimmune disease: A state in which the natural unresponsiveness or tolerance to self terminates. As a result, antibodies or the cells of the immune system react with self constituents and cause disease. Examples of autoimmune diseases are asthma, insulin-dependent diabetes and rheumatoid arthritis.

Bacteria: One-celled microscopic organisms having both plant and animal characteristics ranging from harmless to disease-producing and lethal.

Bactericidal: An agent having the capacity to destroy bacteria.

Beta-carotene: A deep yellow plant pigment that is converted by the body to vitamin A.

Bile salts: Substances which are the end products of cholesterol breakdown and are present in the intestines as aids to fat digestion.

B-lymphocyte: White blood cell of the lymphocyte class, having a single large nucleus. B-lymphocytes are capable of being transformed (after exposure to an antigen) into antibody-producing cells called plasma cells.

Bursa of fabricus: A hindgut lymphoepithelial organ located in the cloaca of birds that controls the function of B-lymphocytes. Removal of this organ in chickens results in a marked deficiency of antibodies and plasma cells.

Calcium: A mineral that is essential for bone and tooth formation; acts as a catalyst in blood clotting; regulates muscle contractibility, including heartbeat and normal nerve transmission; activates enzymes and controls the permeability of the cell membrane to various other nutrients.

Carotene: See Beta-carotene.

Catalase: An iron containing protein (enzyme) which is capable of the removal of hydrogen peroxide, converting it to water and oxygen.

Cell-mediated cytotoxicity: A form of lymphocyte-mediated cytotoxicity in which an effector cell (macrophage, lymphocyte, monocyte) kills an antibody-coated target cell.

Cellular immunity: Immunity in which the participation of macrophages and lymphocytes is predominant.

Cholesterol: A 27 carbon atom derived lipid (fat) or sterol widely distributed in all cells of the body and from which is made: bile salts, adrenal cortical hormones, sex hormones, vitamin D, nerve tissue, etc.

Choline: Metabolite sometimes classified as a B vitamin which participates in fat emulsion and metabolism (as lecithin) and is a constituent of the neuro-transmitter, acetylcholine, which mediates the conduction of messages from nerve tissue to muscles and other tissues.

Chromosome: Rod-like body in the nucleus of a cell which acts as a carrier of genes or units of heredity.

Classic pathway of complement activation: A pathway of activation of the complement proteins which requires the presence of antibodies or antigen-antibody complexes.

Complement system: The primary blood mediator of antigen-antibody reactions. Consists of some twenty distinct plasma proteins capable of interacting with each other and with cell membranes to produce the destruction of an antigen.

Copper: An essential metal for blood synthesis, normal bone formation and the maintenance of myelin (electrical insulation) in the nervous system. Copper is present in two key enzymes, one of which is responsible for 90% of the oxygen consumed by life on earth (cytochrome c oxidase), the other for the degradation of toxic oxygen species produced by metabolism (superoxide dismutase).

Corticosteroids: See cortisol.

Cortisol: Hormones secreted by the cortex of the adrenal gland which appear to suppress the immune system, decrease inflammation and enhance healing.

C-reactive protein: a protein found in the blood of patients with diverse inflammatory diseases which is capable of combining with and promoting the phagocytosis of a variety of bacteria.

Cytostasis: The inhibition of the cellular function of a cancerous cell.

Cytotoxicity: The ability to be poisonous or destructive to a target cell (virus–laden or cancerous).

Cytotoxic T-lymphocyte: A special T-lymphocyte capable of destroying virus or tumor(cancerous)–infected body cells.

Dimethylglycine: An amino acid which is an intermediate compound in the normal metabolism of choline or in the synthesis of the amino acid, glycine, and which has immunopotentiating properties.

DNA (deoxyribonucleic acid): The chemical substance present in the nucleus of every living cell consisting of units whose sequence in a spiral configuration determines the unique genetic makeup of an individual.

Endogenous pyrogen: Protein substances released by white blood cells which produce fever.

Endotoxins: Compounds derived from the cell walls of some microorganisms that have toxic and pyrogenic effects.

Enzyme: A protein-like substance produced by cells which has the power to initiate or accelerate specific biochemical reactions in an organism.

Fatty acids: Constituents of fat. Any of a series of organic acids which react with glycerol to form fats and with metallic bases to form soaps.

Fever: Body temperature which is above the normal.

Folic acid: A vitamin which has the ability to form an enzyme which is capable of transferring carbon atoms in the manufacture of important body chemicals such as DNA, RNA and the amino acid, cystine. Folic acid is essential for the formation of red and white blood cells.

Fungi (fungus): A group of plants that reproduce by spores and have no stems, leaves, roots or chlorophyll, comprising the mushrooms, smuts, molds, puffballs, etc. Microscopic fungi can infect humans.

Gastrointestinal: Having to do with the stomach and intestinal tract and can also include the esophagus.

Gene: A unit occupying a distinct position on a chromosome and having a crucial function in the transmission of a specific characteristic from parent to offspring.

Glycine: The simplest, two-carbon amino acid occurring in proteins.

Granulocyte: See polymorphonuclear phagocyte.

Hair analysis: A method by which hair is dissolved and its mineral constituents are determined.

Helper T-lymphocyte: A subtype of T-lymphocytes that cooperate with B-lymphocytes in antibody formation.

Histamine: A bioactive amine that causes smooth muscle constriction of human bronchioles (in the lungs) and small blood vessels, increased permeability of capillaries, and increased secretion by nasal and bronchial mucous glands. The substance responsible for the symptoms of allergy.

Humoral immunity: Pertaining to molecules in solution in a body fluid (blood) — especially antibodies and the complement proteins.

Hydrogen peroxide: A very unstable compound that decomposes to form water and oxygen. It is also bactericidal.

Hydrolytic enzyme: An enzyme which produces a chemical reaction resulting in the rupture of a covalent bond with addition of the elements of water.

Hydroxyl radical: The univalent radical consisting of one atom of oxygen and one atom of hydrogen (OH). It is especially toxic to cell membranes.

Hyperplasia: An increase in the size of a tissue or organ resulting from proliferation of cells or the development of additional tissue of which the organ is composed, but excluding tumor formation.

Immune complex: An antigen-antibody complex or an antigen-antibody-complement complex.

Immunocompetence: A condition of the immune system where it is able to produce a successful immune response.

Immunocompromised: See immunodeficiency.

Immunodeficiency: A condition of the immune system where it is unable to produce a sufficient immune response.

Immunogen: A substance that when introduced into a human stimulates the immune response.

Immunoglobulin: A protein that functions as an antibody. See antibody.

Immunostimulatory: A condition, substance or substances that stimulate the initiation of the immune response.

Immunosuppression: See immunodeficiency.

Incubate: To maintain under conditions favoring optimal growth or development. To maintain the period between exposure to an infectious disease and the appearance of symptoms.

Inflammation (inflammatory): A localized reaction to infection or injury characterized by heat, redness, swelling and pain.

Interferon: A group of proteins elaborated by infected body cells that protect noninfected cells from viral infection.

Iodine: A crystalline element of the halogen group which is necessary for the formation of the thyroid hormones.

Iron: A mineral which is involved in the transport of oxygen as a constituent of hemoglobin. Iron is also contained in the enzymes, catalase and peroxidase.

Isobutyl Nitrite: See Amyl Nitrite. Isobutyl Nitrite is similar to Amyl Nitrite.

K cells: A special lymphocyte 'killer' cell responsible for antibody-dependent cell-mediated cytotoxicity. See also cytotoxicity.

L-Arginine: See Arginine.

Leukocyte: A white blood cell. See polymorphonuclear leukocyte.

Leukocyte pyrogen: See endogenous pyrogen.

Lipoprotein: A particle which is a combination of fats and protein and is responsible for transporting fats and cholesterol through the blood stream.

L-Lysine: See lysine.

Lymph nodes: Any of the nodular bodies of spongy tissue found in the system of lymphatic vessels usually at the juncture of major lymphatic tracts which serve as traps for foreign invaders and antigens.

Lymphocyte (T & B): A white blood cell with a single large nucleus and a small rim of cytoplasm.

Lymphoma: A general term for growth of new tissue in the lymphatic system. Included in this general group is Hodgkins disease, lymphosarcoma and malignant sarcoma.

Lyse (lysis): The process of cell destruction by rupture of the membrane.

Lysine: A basic, six-carbon amino acid which is found in proteins.

Lysozyme: A protein enzyme present in tears, saliva and nasal secretions that reduces the local concentration of susceptible bacteria.

Macrophage: Phagocytic mononuclear white blood cells that are derived from bone marrow monocytes and sub-serve accessory roles in cellular immunity. See also monocyte.

Magnesium: A mineral which is essential for the normal metabolism of calcium and phosphorus. Magnesium is an activator for the enzymes of carbohydrate and amino acid metabolism and aids in the conduction of nerve impulses.

Metabolism: The aggregate of physical and chemical processes by which the body converts assimilated materials into living tissue, energy and waste.

Microbe: A microscopic organism, especially a disease-producing bacterium.

Microenvironment: The environment surrounding micro-organisms or living cells.

Microgram: One millionth of a gram or one thousandth of a milligram.

Microorganism: An organism visible only in an optical or electron microscope, as a bacterium, protozoan or virus.

Milligram: One thousandth of a gram.

Monocyte: A white blood cell that differs from a lymphocyte by having much more cytoplasm surrounding a large fetus-shaped nucleus. Macrophages are large monocytes.

Mononuclear phagocyte: A monocyte or macrophage. See monocyte.

Mucociliary escalator: A system which, by the whip-like

action of cilia (tiny hair–like projections), transports microorganisms and foreign material to the oropharynx (mouth and throat) from the respiratory tract.

Mycobacteria: A genus of acid–fast bacteria which includes the causative organisms of tuberculosis and leprosy.

Myeloperoxidase: An enzyme present within phagocytic cells which catalyzes peroxidation and destruction of microorganisms.

Natural killer cells (NK cells): Small white blood cells of the lymphocyte class capable of killing a wide variety of tumor cells and other cell lines which does not require the presence of antibody and is not inhibited by immune complexes.

Nuclei (nucleus): A complex spheroidal body found in plant and animal cells which is essential for the vital activities of the cell such as growth and reproduction.

Nucleic acids: Constituents of DNA. See DNA.

Pantothenic acid: An essential B vitamin for humans. As a constituent of coenzyme A in the citric acid cycle, pantothenic acid is required for energy production from fats, carbohydrates and proteins. Pantothenic acid is involved in the production of the nerve transmitter, acetylcholine, and in the biosynthesis of blood and the adrenal gland proteins.

Parasites: Any of a group of microscopic one–celled animals such as amoeba or *Pneumocystis carinii* which cause infection in humans.

Peroxidase: See myeloperoxidase.

Phagocyte: A white blood cell that is capable of ingesting particulate matter including viruses and bacteria.

Phagocytosis: The process by which white blood cells engulf particulate matter and microorganisms.

Plasma cell: A transformed B-lymphocyte which produces antibodies.

Pneumocystis carinii pneumonia: Pneumonia caused by a protozoan parasite. See parasite.

Polymorphonuclear leukocyte: A white blood cell capable of phagocytosis which has its nucleus in clumps connected by strands of chromatin making this cell capable of slipping through and out of the blood stream. Also called a granulocyte.

Pyridoxine (vitamin B_6): A vitamin which forms a coenzyme that participates in nearly all chemical reactions involving amino acids. Vitamin B_6 is necessary for the conversion of the amino acid, tryptophane, to niacin and the conversion of the fat acid, linoleic acid, to arachidonic acid.

Pyrogen: See endogenous pyrogen.

Receptor: An area on the membrane of a cell for adherence or communication of various chemicals or substances such as antigens, antibodies or complement proteins.

Remission: Abatement of a symptom, pain or disease.

Riboflavin (vitamin B_2): A member of the B-complex

family of vitamins necessary for the transfer of hydrogen ions during energy metabolism.

Saturated fat: A fat in which all of the carbon atoms in its structure are linked by single bonds. Examples of saturated fat are butter, tallow and coconut oil.

Selenium: A mineral named after the moon goddess, Selene, which has powerful antioxidant abilities. Selenium is a constituent of the enzyme, glutathione peroxidase, which degrades hydrogen peroxide to water and oxygen as well as assisting to maintain cell membrane integrity. See also antioxidant.

Seminal plasma: The male ejaculate which contains sperm and other concretions designed to facilitate the movement of sperm.

SGOT: An enzyme generally found in the liver and heart muscle and which is liberated into the blood stream if there is disease or damage to these organs.

Spleen: A large lymphoid organ located in the upper left quadrant of the abdomen which contains large populations of lymphocytes.

Stem cell: A bone marrow cell from which most white and red blood cells originate.

Suppressor T-lymphocyte: A subset of T-lymphocytes that suppresses antibody synthesis by B-lymphocytes or inhibits other cellular immune reactions by effector T-lymphocytes.

Synergistically (synergism): The mutually reinforcing action of separate substances, organs or agents which together produce an effect greater than that of all of the components acting separately.

Target cell: An infected or cancerous cell that is being lysed or destroyed by a cytotoxic cell or antigen–antibody–complement action.

Thymic hormones: Chemical substances produced by the thymus gland which have various effects on T-lymphocytes.

Thymus: The lymphoid gland located in the chest behind the breastbone which is responsible for the differentiation of T-lymphocytes.

T-lymphocyte: A thymus-derived white blood cell that participates in a variety of cell-mediated immune reactions.

Tocopherols: See Vitamin E.

Toxic metals: Metals such as lead, mercury or cadmium which cause adverse effects from their accumulation in body tissues.

Trachea: The windpipe. The cylindrical cartilaginous tube, $4\frac{1}{2}$ inches long, from the larynx to the bronchial tubes.

Triglyceride: Three fatty acids (either saturated or unsaturated or both) joined to a central three-carbon chain. The fats we see in nature and have on our bodies.

Tumor: An autonomous, new growth of tissue forming an abnormal mass which performs no physical function. It develops independent of, and unrestricted by normal laws of growth and morphogenesis. A tumor may be either benign or cancerous.

Unsaturated fat or fatty acid: A fat having double bonds between some of its carbon atoms. Examples of unsaturated fats are safflower oil, soybean oil, peanut oil and sesame oil. Generally, unsaturated fats are liquid at room temperature.

Very low density lipoprotein (VLDL): The major blood transporter for triglycerides which is formed in the liver. See also lipoprotein.

Vitamin A: An oil or lipid soluble vitamin which is a constituent of the pigments involved in the visual process, which maintains normal epithelial tissue, which provides for normal bone and teeth development and which promotes normal growth.

Vitamin B_2: See riboflavin.

Vitamin B_6: See pyridoxine.

Vitamin B_{12}: A B-complex vitamin that is involved in the metabolism of single carbon units and participates in DNA synthesis, myelin (nerve insulation) synthesis and red blood cell maturation.

Vitamin C: See ascorbic acid.

Vitamin E: An oil or lipid soluble vitamin that participates as an antioxidant, protects unsaturated fatty acids and vitamin A from oxidation, participates in the synthesis of hemoglobin and maintains cell membrane integrity.

Virus: Any of a class of ultramicroscopic disease-producing microorganisms capable of reproduction only within specific living systems.

VLDL: See very low density lipoprotein.

Zinc: A mineral which is a member of a large number of enzymes with such diverse activities as maintaining the acid–base balance of the body, participating in the metabolism of proteins and nucleic acids, regulating the hormone, insulin, and stimulating wound healing.

PART ONE

Nutrition and Immunity: An Intimate Relationship

Generally, in order to produce some disease in an organism there must be some threat from the environment. Whether or not humans succumb to this threat is a function of their capacity to repel this external bombardment. Health or disease, then, is the result of an environmental challenge imposed upon an organism which is either resistant or susceptible.[1,2]

Prevention, and even prediction, of disease can be facilitated by two processes, each of which is equally important: remove whatever is causing the disease condition (environmental challenge) or increase resistance to the disease and thereby lower susceptibility.

In many, if not all, cases it is nearly impossible to remove an infectious agent from the environment. In some diseases the infectious agent may not even be identified or may not be an infectious agent at all. With the aforementioned in mind what seems most important is to consider how to improve resistance to disease.

On a global scale undernutrition (or malnutrition) is the most common cause of a deficiency of the immune response. It has long been accepted that undernutrition contributes to increased illness and death, particularly from infectious diseases. Careful clinical observations and epidemiological surveys (studies to determine disease risk factors) have established the intimate relationship, probably a causal one, between nutritional deficiency and infection.[3,4,5,6,7]

The prevalence, severity and pattern of infections in poorly nourished individuals mimic the characteristic manifestations of primary immunodeficiency disorders. For example, infections with organisms such as parasites, viruses, fungi and bacteria are seen both in primary defects of the immune apparatus and in nutrition-related impairment of the immune system.[4,5,8,9] Diseases caused by parasites such as *Pneumocystis carinii*, which results in pneumonia, were first described in malnourished, institutionalized children in Europe after World War II and persisted as a problem until the children's nutritional state improved.[9] The incidence of measles is more prevalent, severe and prolonged in malnourished children.[5,10] Fungal infections from organisms such as *Candida*, bacterial and viral diarrhea and infections resulting from surgical procedures increase in undernutrition.[5] Herpes virus infections, tuberculosis, intestinal parasites, malaria, pertussis, diphtheria, influenza, small pox, tetanus, poliomyelitis, *Staphylococcus* and *Streptococcus* infections and even syphilis are influenced by nutritional status.[5] Finally, it is known that many viruses tend to persist indefinitely in a dormant state in tissues, especially if viruses are encoded into the chromosomes, or nucleic acids, of cells, and express themselves when favorable conditions arise, that is, when the body's defenses are low (poor health).[11]

Nutritional disorders are particularly common in underdeveloped countries, but it has now been established that undernutrition occurs in all segments of all populations including hospitalized patients in the

United States, Canada and other industrialized countries.[3,4,5]

The increased susceptibility of elderly people to infectious and cancerous diseases appears to be a consequence of senescence of the immune system[12], yet a study of the effects of nutritional supplementation for just eight weeks on the nutrition and immunocompetence of elderly persons showed that nutritional support increased immune responses.[13]

PART TWO

The Department of Defense: The White Army, The Immune Response, The Red Army and Other Soldiers

A normally functioning immune system is an effective defense against foreign infectious agents and against body cells that have become cancerous.[14] The immune system is complex, but it is capable of exerting multiple effects which are expressed by only a few distinct cell types. Depending on the momentary needs of the body, the immune regulatory mechanism may amplify a given immunogenic response or diminish it. The complex organization of the cellular and molecular components of the immune system allows flexibility of response so that the body is not limited to only one possible pathway in response to foreign invasion or disease. This helps to insure the ultimate destruction of the invader or disease.

The immune regulatory mechanisms are genetically controlled. In humans these genes are located on the short arm of chromosome six and regulate such functions as interactions between the cellular components of the immune system (macrophages and T- and B-lymphocytes), whether or not an individual is capable of responding to certain antigens or immunogens (substances that induce an immune response when introduced into the body), susceptibility to disease, the production of chemical mediators that regulate the actions of the cells involved in immune responses, susceptibility to allergic and autoimmune diseases, and the structure and function of antibodies.[14,15]

The White Army

The major cellular components of the immune system (cellular immunity) are white blood cells: the macrophages and the lymphocytes.

MACROPHAGES
During an inflammatory process or infection, leukocytes (white blood cells) engulf microorganisms by a process called phagocytosis. There are two types of phagocytes (cells which engulf): polymorphonuclear leukocytes (the nuclei of these cells are lobulated enabling them to squeeze through blood vessel walls in order to reach infected tissues) which circulate in the blood and migrate to sites of inflammation, and mononuclear phagocytes (the nuclei of these cells appear as a single ovoid or elongated worm-like structure) which are found circulating in the blood and fixed or stationary in tissues (such as the liver, bone, lungs, joints and lymph nodes). These also accumulate at sites of inflammation.[16,17] Both of these cell types are capable of recognizing, ingesting and digesting foreign particles. These cells were originally termed macrophages because of their phagocytic ability. Today the term macrophage is reserved for the large mononuclear phagocyte, and the term granulocyte is applied to the polymorphonuclear leukocyte. All of these cells are produced in the bone marrow from a common cell type, the stem cell. The

most prominent functional property of the macrophage and the granulocyte is their ability to recognize foreign or damaged materials.[16]

Once foreign matter (bacteria, viruses, etc.) has been ingested, the macrophage kills and digests its prey. This is accomplished by producing toxic substances made from oxygen, such as hydrogen peroxide or hydroxyl radical.[16,18,19,20] In addition to these reactive or toxic species of oxygen, the antimicrobial effects of hydrogen peroxide are augmented by chlorine or iodine ions in the presence of the proteinaceous enzymes, myeloperoxidase or catalase. Vitamin C may also act along with hydrogen peroxide to kill ingested microorganisms.[20,21] After macrophages have inactivated their engulfed meal they can produce over forty hydrolytic enzymes which act in an acid medium to digest the ingested material.[16]

Macrophages may also inhibit the growth of, or kill, cancerous cells by releasing the previously mentioned toxic species of oxygen; by depriving the cancer of the essential amino acid, L–Arginine, or by causing the cancerous cells to lyse if they have been coated with antibodies.[16,21,22]

More than fifty chemical products which macrophages secrete have also been identified. The role of macrophages as secretory cells may be just as important in their interaction with metabolism as is their role as phagocytic cells. For instance, macrophages produce a number of enzymes which they use not only in defense systems but also in the mechanism of the coagulation and clotting of blood.[16] Macrophages produce proteins involved in fat transport and may play an important role in the regulation of triglyceride and cholesterol metabolism.[16] The macrophage secretes virtually all of the components of the complement system (*see page 47*), factors promoting proliferation of T- and B-lymphocytes, interferon and a factor which promotes fever production (endogenous pyrogen).[16,20]

Macrophages are capable of either enhancing or suppressing the viability of lymphocytes. They produce factors which activate T-lymphocytes and, like a well-trained butler, they process and present immunogenic molecules and foreign infecting agents to the lymphocyte.[11,14,16]

LYMPHOCYTES

There are two major types of lymphocytes, B- and T-lymphocytes. T-lymphocytes can further be subdivided by their regulatory and effector functions. Regulatory T-lymphocytes include the helper/inducer T-lymphocyte and the suppressor T-lymphocyte, both of which either amplify or suppress the response of other T-lymphocytes or of B-lymphocytes.[14,23,24,25] Failure of the suppressor T-lymphocyte may result in the unchecked activity of the helper/inducer T-lymphocyte function with the result of the immune apparatus being directed toward the body's own native cells which may cause such autoimmune diseases as rheumatoid arthritis, asthma or juvenile insulin-dependent diabetes.[26] Activated T-lymphocytes also produce chemicals which attract, activate and trap macrophages in inflammatory tissue.[11]

Effector T-lymphocytes (cytotoxic T-lymphocytes) are responsible for rejection of foreign tissue grafts (such as kidney and heart transplants) and cancerous tumors and elimination of virus infected body cells.[14,25] The suppressor and cytotoxic T-lymphocytes actually belong to the same subpopulation of T-lymphocytes and the only way to distinguish them is to perform tests for their individual functions.[27]

T-lymphocytes are manufactured in the bone marrow and then migrate to a gland located in the chest, the thymus gland (hence the 'T'). The T-lymphocyte 'matures' in the thymus and receives functional competence there. When T-lymphocytes become adults they are exported to the spleen, lymph nodes and blood. The optimal health of the thymus gland is essential to correct T-lymphocyte differentiation.[24,25] This gland reaches its maximum size at birth and decreases with age.[12]

Properly activated T-lymphocytes induce or suppress B-lymphocytes. Activated B-lymphocytes transform into large antibody (immunoglobulin) producing cells, plasma cells, and memory B-lymphocytes. The purpose of memory B-lymphocytes is for the production of rapid antibody responses upon re-exposure to the same antigen that elicited the initial response.[11,14] Antibodies are Y-shaped proteins which are capable of attaching onto foreign invading micro-organisms or tumor cells, thereby either blocking their attachment to body cells or allowing for the complement system to destroy the invader or macrophages or cytotoxic lymphocytes to either lyse or engulf and destroy the invader.[20,21] The antibody and complement systems are considered to be the humoral (molecules in solution in a body fluid) components of the immune system.

B-lymphocytes are so named because they are functionally similar to the antibody-producing cells located in a lymphoid organ present in birds, the bursa of Fabricus. Even though no equivalent structure has been found in mammals, the 'bursa equivalent' or 'B' terminology remains.[25] The origin of B-lymphocytes appears to be bone marrow or the fetal liver.[11,25] B-lymphocytes may be found in the spleen, lymph nodes, trachea, small intestine, vaginal mucosa and tonsils.[25]

NATURAL KILLER (NK) CELLS AND K CELLS

Natural killer cells are lymphocytes, but they are different from cytotoxic T-lymphocytes. Cytotoxic T-lymphocytes are immunologically specific whereas NK cells can kill other cells across organ, strain and species barriers.[28] Natural killer cells are characterized by their ability to destroy a wide variety of cell types especially cancerous lymphomas and tumor cells.

K cells are also lymphocytes but they require the presence of antibodies on the surface of their target cells. The antibody serves 'to bridge' the K cell to the target cell, and thus mediate destruction of the target cell.[28] K cell mediated cytotoxicity may contribute to the eradication of some cancers, but its exact role in body defenses has been difficult to establish.[28]

The Immune Response

Whenever the body encounters a foreign intruder such as a virus or bacterium, classically the macrophages and lymphocytes interact resulting in the production of specific antibodies which combine with the invader or antigen. Another group of proteins in the blood, complement, attaches itself, too. Complement then orchestrates the final rupture and destruction of the antigen.[11,14,29] Cellular debris and complexes resulting from the action of antibodies and complement are then ingested and digested by the phagocytes. With the disappearance of the antigen, antibody synthesis halts and there is a decline of antibody presence in the blood. The body's initial, or primary, response to an antigen is of less magnitude than a secondary response evoked by reexposure to the same antigen. In a secondary response there is a higher rate and longer duration of antibody synthesis, and a slower rate of decline after the antigen has been suppressed. The capacity for the secondary response can persist for many years which may account for the long-lasting immunity against some viral infections. Even after antibodies to a specific antigen are no longer detectable, reexposure to small amounts of antigen can evoke prompt elaboration of large amounts of highly efficient antibody.[11]

The Red Army

Traditionally it has been assumed that red blood cells have only a single mission in life: to transport oxygen throughout the body. White blood cells which are fewer in number seem to be more warrior-like, prowling through the blood stream and destroying foreign invaders. If these white blood cells were not effective no one would survive. The efficiency of this system is surprising, since these complex defense maneuvers are accomplished only by white blood cells which account for less than one per cent of the total blood volume. It may be that red blood cells, which far outnumber white blood cells, may also help defend the body.[30]

Over fifty years ago researchers first noticed that red

cells adhere to some single-celled parasites and in the 1950s it was demonstrated that red cells adhere to antigen–antibody–complement complexes (immune complexes) and that the presence of the red cell's adherence augments the engulfment of the antigen by white cells. When both red and white blood cells are mixed with bacteria and antibody and incubated, after one hour 95 per cent of the bacteria disappear. When the same mixture is incubated but without the red cells, all of the bacteria remain.[30]

Red blood cells also interact with the complement system and have receptors on their surfaces for complement proteins exactly the same as the receptors on white blood cells.[29,30] Red blood cells account for 95 per cent of all the receptors for the complement component C3b. Since an antigen–antibody–complement complex collides at random with white blood cells (the collision is essential for the removal of the complex), the complex has a thousand times more chances to collide with a red cell than with a white cell. This suggests that red cells may play the major role in the initial destruction of foreign invaders.

It has also been discovered that there are two blood chemicals which regulate the adherence of red cells, an inhibitor and a promoter, which suggests that this activity is being methodically regulated by the body.[30] Red cells adhere not only to antigen and immune complexes but also to T–lymphocytes which may mean that red cells function in much the same way as macrophages in presenting antigens to T–lymphocytes.[30]

The presence of the enzyme, peroxidase, on red blood cell surfaces was discovered in 1965. This property was thought to be confined to macrophages. Peroxidase may enable the red cell to damage the antigen to which it adheres. The parts of the red cell surface membrane that adhere to antigens are the same areas where the 'killer enzyme', peroxidase, is the most active.[30]

Some cancer patients have been observed to have a decrease in red cell immune adherence and the adherence of red cells to T-lymphocytes is depressed in cancer patients and returns to normal if the cancer goes into remission.[30] Patients with the autoimmune disease, systemic lupus erythematosis, which is characterized by a buildup of immune complexes and antibodies, have very low red cell immune activity.

Other Soldiers

THE COMPLEMENT SYSTEM
The complement system consists of at least twenty chemically and immunologically distinct blood proteins capable of interacting with each other, with antibodies and with cell membranes. The individual proteins of the system are normally present in the circulation as inactive molecules and must be activated in sequence under appropriate conditions in order for a complement reaction to progress.[29] Activation is not a single event, but a dynamic process allowing the proteins to become interacting members of an integrated system.

Acting like master sergeants at military recruitment centers, complement is able to enlist the aid of lymphocytes, phagocytes and red blood cells. Complement also interacts with white blood cells in the destruction of parasitic organisms and the activation of allergic responses.[29]

And, as if the whole immune system weren's complex enough already, there are two parallel, but entirely independent, pathways leading to the terminal biological function of the complement sequence.

The complement system is the primary mediator of antigen–antibody reactions and is activated by antigen–antibody complexes, antibodies and nonimmunological substances such as proteins formed from inflammation, cell membranes and DNA.[29] Complement functions by progressive accumulation on the cell membrane of the target cell which results in membrane damage via opening a channel to the interior through which water flows causing the cell membrane to swell and burst.[11,29]

In the process of complement accumulation segments are broken off the main proteins. These segments possess the capacity to attract macrophages and induce inflammation which isolates the area of infection.

DEFENSES AT BODY SURFACES

In order for a foreign invader to produce infection it must breach a barrier of surface defenses which operate wherever intact body tissues confront the environment. Lysozyme, a proteinaceous enzyme present in tears, nasal secretions and saliva, reduces local concentrations of susceptible bacteria. Stomach acidity prevents some bacteria, viruses and parasites from reaching the intestine. Acidity of the skin and vaginal secretions retards infections and seminal plasma contains proteins and zinc which possess potent bactericidal activity.[11,20] Fatty acids and bile salts in the intestine are inhibitory for many microorganisms. The non-disease producing bacteria that normally inhabit the body produce fatty acids and stimulate the production of antibodies, both of which retard bacterial colonization.[11,20]

It must be realized that simple processes such as sneezing, salivation, tearing, coughing, defecating, urinating and diarrhea also aid in the removal of potentially disease-causing microorganisms from the body. The mucociliary escalator of the respiratory tract brings foreign material to the mouth and throat where it may be coughed out or swallowed and excreted through the bowl.[20]

INTERFERON

Interferon is a family of proteins produced by body cells in response to a variety of stimuli, including viral infections. These proteins exhibit antiviral activity by inducing cells to produce other proteins which interfere with viral replication. Additionally, interferons inhibit the growth of certain cancerous cells.[20,31,32] Interferon is produced by, and released from, cells early in the course of viral infection and is available much earlier than antibodies are. Interferon's antiviral activity may be transferred to neighboring cells, without continued presence, by an unknown mechanism.[20] Interferon increases white blood cell toxicity and augments the destructive activity of natural killer (NK) cells and cytotoxic T-lymphocytes.[20,28]

FEVER

The occurrence of fever in infectious diseases is so common that its presence generally indicates a search for an invading microorganism. However, the true significance of fever remains uncertain.[20] Notwithstanding, there is some evidence that it operates in body defenses. Macrophages demonstrate their maximum ingesting activity at temperatures above normal. During fever there is a decrease in the circulating level of iron and a reduction in the ability of bacteria to concentrate iron which they must have in order to grow and reproduce.[20]

The stimulus to fever production results from the presence of a circulating protein known as leukocyte pyrogen or endogenous pyrogen. This substance is produced by phagocytes and macrophages in response to microbial agents, antigen–antibody complexes and bacterial toxins.[20]

PART THREE

Fortification of the Immune System: Manufacturing Steel Dolls

It is as though I had on a table three dolls, one of glass, another of celluloid, and a third of steel, and I chose to hit the three dolls with a hammer, using equal strength. The first doll would break, the second doll would scar and the third would emit a pleasant musical note.[33]

In Part One it was proposed that the prevention of disease could be facilitated by increasing resistance and thereby lowering susceptibility. What now remains is to consider how to improve resistance to disease or how to make a steel doll (resistant body) out of a glass doll (susceptible body) or at least turn the glass doll into celluloid (partially resistant body).

Diet

The first ingredient in the steel doll recipe must be adequate, high quality protein. The highest quality proteins which maintain efficiency for humans are the animal proteins: eggs, cheese, cottage cheese and meats (beef, lamb, poultry, pork and fish). In order to maintain drug and foreign chemical detoxification functions of the body at their maximum, 20 per cent of the caloric intake should be high quality protein.[34] T-lymphocytes are profoundly affected by protein deficiency and skimping here even marginally can reduce T-lymphocyte function by 35 per cent,[3] a level which may be expected to enhance the risk and severity of infection.[5]

When protein deficiency is combined with a less than adequate intake of calories, all lymphoid organs (tonsils, thymus, spleen, lymph nodes, etc.) atrophy and there is a decrease in thymic hormones.[4] Blood samples from individuals with protein-calorie malnutrition contain increased amounts of chemicals known to inhibit immune responses, such as cortisol, endotoxins and antigen-antibody complexes and C-reactive protein.[4,5] Individuals with protein-calorie malnutrition have a high incidence of infection, particularly with mycobacteria, viruses and fungi, and show low levels of lymphocytes in their blood. Interferon production is lower than normal.[4,5] In many cases of protein-calorie malnutrition there is an actual increase in the production of some antibodies, while others are depressed. With severe protein-calorie malnutrition there is a decrease in B-lymphocytes with reduction in all antibody levels.[4,5] The activity of several enzyme systems responsible for killing bacteria is reduced. A number of the protein components of the complement system are also reduced.[4,5] Patients with protein-calorie malnutrition have a pronounced reduction in the proportion of helper T-lymphocytes and a moderately reduced proportion of suppressor T-lymphocytes and cytotoxic T-lymphocytes.[4,5] Protein-calorie malnutrition leads to a decrease in the number of red blood cells, thus lowering the number of soldiers in the red army.

Diets high in protein have been shown to enhance

cancerous tumor rejection and cell–mediated cytotoxicity in animals.[4]

One really need not be concerned with contracting cancer from eating meat since a number of studies have absolved meat in this regard[35,36,37,38] and neither are hormones in meat when they do appear of any consequence.[39] It should be noted, however, that fish is a known initiator of human gastro–intestinal cancers.[38] Meats in general are a good source of iron and red meat is one of the best sources of available zinc that exists.[40] The importance of iron and zinc will emerge later on. Protein cannot be overemphasized especially when one considers that antibodies and complement are composed entirely of protein and enzymes that white blood cells use to poison and digest microbes are proteins. Adequate intake of protein foods for both adult men and women could be obtained from no less than three cups of cottage cheese per day or twelve ounces of poultry, lean beef, lamb, fish or lean pork. If only eggs were consumed as the protein source about fourteen would be needed on a daily basis, and if only milk were consumed three quarts would be needed daily.

Research regarding the relationship of fats to immunity indicates that deficiencies of essential unsaturated fats impair cellular immunity, but that excess amounts also result in impairment.[3,4,5] Linoleic acid and arachidonic acid, two polyunsaturated fatty acids, have been shown to be required nutrients and their absence results in reduced antibody production.[4,5] Determining the exact amount of essential unsaturated fats that is optimal is particularly difficult in humans, but erring on the side of excess should be avoided since immunosuppression and cancer promotion can be elicited at least temporarily by an excess of fats of the unsaturated variety.[4,5,41,42] Unsaturated fats are those oils such as safflower or sunflower which are liquid at room temperature and are usually used in deep frying or on salads. They should not be heated and their intake should be accompanied by vitamin E. Drug and foreign chemical detoxification functions of the liver, lungs, kidneys and small intestines also require these unsaturated fats.[43] Vegetable oils probably should be limited to two tablespoons or less per day.

Research on saturated fats, the fat which appears on meats and is in butter and coconut oil, is sparse but indicates that there is no interference from moderate amounts of this nutrient on either the immune response or drug detoxification functions where tested in animals.[43,44,45] However, high levels of saturated fat in the blood stream may be associated with decreased resistance to infections and cancers that have been transplanted onto animals.[4,5] This effect could be explained by the fact that saturated fat also contains unsaturated fat, and that experimentally high fat diets produce a blood factor which inhibits T-lymphocytes and which has been identified as a lipoprotein (a transporter or delivery vehicle for fat).[4] When human lymphocytes are cultured in the presence of even very high levels of fat, immune responses are not suppressed as long as a balance between unsaturated and saturated fat is maintained.[4] It must be remembered that fatty acids are components of tissue and body fluids and do have antibacterial effects and are capable of killing some foreign invaders.[11]

Cholesterol may be immunosuppressive only when the blood shows abnormally high levels of this nutrient.[4,5] Actually, since less than 20 per cent of the cholesterol in the diet ends up in the blood[46] there is no need to consciously decrease the amount of dietary cholesterol in the context of immune responsiveness. There is evidence that in some cases a high blood cholesterol may even facilitate T-lymphocyte responses.[4,47,48] Cholesterol is required for successful proliferation of lymphocytes once they have been stimulated.[5,49]

High carbohydrate diets should be avoided because not only do they suppress the drug and foreign chemical detoxification systems of the body,[34] but the resulting increases in blood sugar, especially if prolonged, may impair both phagocyte and lymphocyte function as well as decrease antibody synthesis.[4] High carbohydrate diets also result in increases in blood triglyceride (a blood fat) levels and increased production of the transporting lipoprotein for triglycerides, very low density lipoprotein (VLDL).[50] Very low density lipoprotein specifically inhibits protein and DNA synthesis in lymphocytes.[4] Lowering the intake of carbohydrates can be accomplished by reducing the intake of sweet drinks, sugar, candy, desserts, bread, french fries, pasta, cereal, etc.

Large amounts of vegetables in the diet may affect a normal or immunocompromised individual in two ways. First, the intake of large amounts of vegetables may cause a decrease in some persons in the number of white cells in the blood.[51,52] Second, bacteria and fungi have been found to accompany a high percentage of fresh vegetables.[53] Fresh fruit juices have also been shown to be heavily contaminated.[54] It has been suggested that one way of reducing bacterial and fungal infections in immunocompromised patients is to reduce or eliminate these foods.[55] On the other hand, Brussels sprouts, cabbage and cauliflower have been shown to stimulate the detoxification of drugs and toxic chemicals.[34] Vegetables and fruit should be carefully washed or peeled. Perhaps it might be best to eat most vegetables steamed. Fresh fruits rather than their juices should be consumed. All foods should be obtained in their freshest possible state and prepared with a minimum of cooking except for pork which should be well done. In a person whose immune system is suppressed, all meats including beef should be well cooked.

Vitamins

Deficiencies of certain vitamins greatly affect the immune system and their repletion in a deficient organism greatly improves the immune status.

VITAMIN B_6 (PYRIDOXINE)

Lack of vitamin B_6 appears consistently to inhibit cell-mediated immune functions as well as antibody production.[4,56] Optimal health of the thymus gland is critical to T-lymphocyte function and vitamin B_6 deficiency results in atrophy of both the thymus and spleen.[4,57] Humans subjected to B_6 deficiencies exhibit diminished antibody production[58] and when B_6 deficiency is combined with a pantothetic acid deficiency (another B vitamin) there is no antibody response at all![59] The phagocytic activity of white blood cells is reduced in B_6 deficiency.[4] The range of intake of vitamin B_6 can be from two milligrams to 1,500 milligrams per day and can be adjusted to dream recall, i.e., consume enough to produce memory of dreams. Increasing the amount of protein in the diet calls for an increase in vitamin B_6. As with all other B vitamins, vitamin B_6 should be taken with the entire B-complex family of vitamins. Vitamin B_6 may interfere with the clotting of blood so that those who are anticipating surgery or have bleeding disorders or are taking anticoagulants should use the vitamin cautiously.

PANTOTHENIC ACID

As with vitamin B_6, pantothenic acid deficiencies also result in atrophy and loss of function of the thymus gland.[57] Experimental animals experience reduced antibody formation.[4,60] Humans seem to be most susceptible when there is a combined deficiency of pantothenic acid and vitamin B_6.[59] The range of intake for pantothenic acid can be from four milligrams to 2,000 milligrams per day.

FOLIC ACID

Deficiencies of the B vitamin, folic acid, lead to a decrease in resistance and to impaired lymphocyte functions in both humans and experimental animals.[4,5,61,62] Deficiencies of folic acid result in impaired antibody production.[4] Folic acid is also necessary for the soldiers of the red army, the red blood cells. Folic acid requirements increase when drugs and foreign chemicals are being detoxified and folic acid deficiency results in decreased metabolism of drugs and foreign chemicals.[43] No less than 0.4 milligrams of folic acid should be obtained daily and much more can safely be taken as evidenced by the over-the-counter sale of 5 milligram tablets in other countries. Folic acid supplementation should be accompanied by vitamin B_{12} since folic acid can mask a vitamin B_{12} deficiency.

VITAMIN B_{12} (CYANOCOBALAMIN)
Because of the difficulty in producing a vitamin B_{12} deficiency in experimental animals, few immunological tests have been performed in vitamin B_{12} deficiency states. Those that have been done indicate that vitamin B_{12} is required for proper lymphocyte function.[4,63] Turnover and production of amino acids (protein) and DNA in the soldiers of the white army is dependent upon vitamin B_{12}.[4,64] The production of red blood cells is also vitamin B_{12} dependent. Intake of vitamin B_{12} may range from 3 micrograms to 1,000 or 2,000 micrograms per day. Intake of amounts over 1,000 micrograms helps insure absorption and vitamin B_{12} may depend upon substances produced by the stomach for optimal absorption. Because Vitamin B_{12} occurs reliably only in animal sources, vegetarians should supplement their diets with this vitamin.

VITAMIN B_2 (RIBOFLAVIN)
On an immunological basis, riboflavin deficiency resembles that of pantothenic acid deficiency, with a diminished ability to generate antibodies.[57,65] Intake of vitamin B_2 should be no less than 1.6 milligrams per day and may need to be as high as 500 to 600 milligrams per day in dependency states. Foods which naturally contain most, if not all, of the B-complex vitamins are organ meats, meats in general, eggs, brewer's yeast, wheat germ, milk, cheese and rice polish.

VITAMIN C (ASCORBIC ACID)

Vitamin C occupies a very important position in immune system functions. When human volunteers are fed at least 1,000 milligrams of vitamin C per day, their antibodies and complement proteins are seen to increase.[66] Experimental animals survive induced influenza virus infections with greater success if they are treated with vitamin C before they are inoculated.[67] Guinea pigs which are kept vitamin C deficient have decreased T–lymphocyte numbers, but if they are given excess vitamin C the T–lymphocyte numbers are increased.[68] Vitamin C is utilized when white blood cells engulf bacteria, viruses and cellular debris[4,69] and supplementation of vitamin C improves the ability of white blood cells to increase the speed with which they get to infected areas.[70] Macrophages combine hydrogen peroxide with ascorbic acid, metal ions, antibody, complement and lysozyme to kill ingested bacteria.[4,20,21] Recent information suggests that vitamin C influences the ability of different body cells (skin, lung) to effect a substantial production of the antiviral agent, interferon.[71,72,73] The thymus gland also requires vitamin C for its optimal activity in producing T–lymphocytes.[74] Experimental animals kept in a vitamin C deficient state experience decreases in their ability to detoxify drugs and foreign chemicals on the order of 50 to 65 per cent.[43] Vitamin C also inhibits the conversion of many chemicals to cancer–causing substances, particularly the nitrates and nitrites used as food preservatives in processed meats (ham, bacon, cold cuts, etc.).[43,75]

Increased losses of vitamin C accompany infection and fever.[76] Histamine (a bioactive amine produced from the amino acid, histidine) which often accompanies inflammation and especially allergic reactions, has been demonstrated to be immunosuppressive.[31] Vitamin C functions as an antihistamine and blocks the enzymes which produce these amines.[77]

How much vitamin C can be tolerated by humans? Foraging gorillas get between 4,000 and 5,000 milligrams of vitamin C per day, but they have to eat 45 to 50 pounds of forest to maintain that intake. Fortunately for humans, vitamin C can be gotten in tablets. It can also be obtained in forms that are not acidic for those with sensitive stomachs. Nutritionists can determine the proper level of vitamin C intake by testing for its presence either in the blood (which can be done for most vitamins) or by a simple pain-free test done on the tongue. The intake can be adjusted individually according to need. The range may be from as little as 60 milligrams per day to as high as 100,000 milligrams per day in unusual cases.[77] Natural sources for vitamin C include all fresh, growing foods. The richest sources are citrus fruits, guavas, ripe bell peppers and pimientos as well as the seed pods of wild roses. Tomato juice, cabbage and strawberries are fair sources. Fresh calves' liver has as much as an orange. Much of the vitamin C in foods is lost if they are stored at room temperature or are soaked or boiled and the water discarded. Frozen foods that are thawed lose their vitamin C within an hour after defrosting.

VITAMIN A

Experimental animals that are deficient in vitamin A experience a decrease in their number of circulating lymphocytes[78] and have lowered resistance to viruses as well as decreased thymus gland and spleen weights.[4,79] Vitamin A is necessary for maintaining the functional integrity of the skin and membranes which line the lungs and digestive tract. Enzymes which can destroy bacteria and viruses are reduced in the white blood cells of vitamin A deficient children.[80] Surgery patients who were given 30,000 to 50,000 international units per day of vitamin A for seven days prior to surgery did not exhibit the normal postoperative depression of lymphocyte counts or responsiveness as was seen in an unsupplemented group.[81] Animals which are *not* deficient in vitamin A and are given supplements of this vitamin increase their resistance to various infective agents.[4,82] Vitamin A and synthetic chemicals resembling vitamin A have been shown to inhibit the development of induced cancers of the skin, colon, breast and respiratory tract.[43]

What levels of vitamin A can humans safely ingest? Generally, 50,000 international units of vitamin A may be taken on a daily basis with safety,[83] but when there is a suspicion of liver disease or low protein intake, any supplementation of vitamin A may result in toxicity.[84] Alcohol consumed in association with vitamin A intake that is usually innocuous results in unusual toxicity to the liver.[84] (Don't take vitamin A with an alcoholic beverage.) Symptoms of vitamin A toxicity may include headache, nausea, loss of appetite, stiff neck, face peeling, lip fissuring and elevation of blood vitamin A levels (except in protein deficiency) and elevation of the liver enzyme, SGOT.[83] Natural sources for vitamin A include liver and fish liver oils, egg yolks, butter and cream. Vitamin A can also be gotten from carotene, a yellow pigment found in carrots, apricots, yams, all green vegetables, cantaloupe, papaya, peaches and sea-weeds. Carotene is also available as beta–carotene sold in capsules. Beta-carotene appears to have none of the possible toxic side effects of increased amounts of veget-ables or vitamin A and large amounts of carotene will not lead to large amounts of vitamin A in blood or to the symptoms of vitamin A toxicity.[51,85] It will, how-ever, lend a yellowish-orange cast to the skin which is harmless.

VITAMIN E (TOCOPHEROLS)
Astonishingly, nearly all of the studies that have been done with vitamin E in connection to immune function have been done using Vitamin E in excess dosages. Experimental animals given excess vitamin E in their food increase their resistance to infection and exhibit a four-fold increase in survival rate.[86,87] Antibodies increase two- to three-fold in animals fed excesses of vitamin E_4,[88] and when made deficient, these animals produced no antibodies at all![89] Vitamin E is involved in the T–lymphocyte stimulation of B–lymphocytes and may be able to stimulate B–lymphocytes without T-lymphocyte intervention in the presence of a normal thymus gland.[90] Similar to B_6 and pantothenic acid, the immunostimulatory effects of vitamin E are enhanced if administered together with the trace min-eral, selenium, in modest excess.[3,5,91] Eight-week-old pigs have been plied with as much as 100,000 interna-tional units of vitamin E daily,[88] but this is far in excess of what humans should consume. Amounts of 800 to 1,600 international units per day have been observed to improve the immune response in humans[87] and appear to be the appropriate dosage although more may be

required in some cases. Since vitamin E is stored over the entire body rather than in the liver, it has extremely low or no toxicity. Vitamin E is required to protect vitamin A from oxidation and may enhance the effect of vitamin A.[92] In actuality there are eight forms of vitamin E and the greatest antioxidant effects (prevents damage from oxygen) of vitamin E are exhibited when the vitamin is used as 'mixed tocopherols'. When purchased the label will read, 'd-alpha tocopherol from mixed tocopherols'. Natural sources of vitamin E are found in the oils of all grains, nuts and seeds. The vitamin may be lost during exposure to air, heating, freezing and storage.

Those who have high blood pressure should consume vitamin E in very low dosages with careful monitoring especially during stepwise increases in dosages, since vitamin E improves heart muscle tone and may temporarily increase blood pressure. Vitamin E, like vitamin B_6, may interfere with blood clotting, so those anticipating surgery should curtail their use of vitamin E before surgery and those with bleeding disorders or taking anticoagulants should use the vitamin cautiously.

Minerals

The importance of minerals and trace minerals in human nutrition has been appreciated only in the past ten to fifteen years. Prior to this the only time the public concerned itself with zinc or magnesium was in connection with galvanized pipes and automobile wheels. Very recent research has elucidated the critical role that minerals play in nutrition and especially the immune response.

IRON

As a single nutrient iron is of major importance. Iron deficiency is one of the most likely forms of single nutrient deficiency to occur in the absence of any other form of malnutrition and iron has profound effects on immune system functions. Either a lack of iron or an excess may create problems. Bacteria and parasites require adequate quantities of iron in order to grow, reproduce and exert their toxic effects. During infections the availability of iron is limited by moving iron into tissues for storage and binding iron to transport proteins making this mineral unavailable to infectious organisms. Further, the soldiers of the white army are able to restrain bacterial growth by releasing iron-binding proteins which 'steal' the iron from the invading microbe.[4,21,93] Additionally, these iron-binding proteins have direct bacteriostatic effects.[4,21] If dietary protein is lacking these binding proteins cannot be adequtein is lacking these binding proteins cannot be adequately manufactured and should excess iron be taken in such a situation, it may not be bound and more iron will become available to invading organisms thus allowing them to flourish.[4,94] In contrast to iron excess, a deficiency in iron can increase susceptibility to infectious diseases. Iron deficiency produces a decreased number of T- and B-lymphocytes,[95] but iron therapy reverses this effect.[96] Iron deficiency affects the function of macrophages and granulocytes by reducing their ability to kill microbes once they have entered the interior of the white blood cell.[4,5,97] Adequate iron is a crucial factor for the activity of enzymes that produce substances (the toxic species of oxygen and hydroxyl radical) that are poisonous to microbes.[4,5,18] These changes in the immune response can be noted with as little as a ten per cent decrease in dietary iron.[4]

Iron is also necessary for the proper 'feeding' of the red army and its deficiency results in a decrease in both the integrity and number of red blood cells. Iron is required for the drug and foreign chemical detoxifying mechanisms of the intestinal tract.[43]

Although steel dolls may be made of iron it is probably not advisable to race to the nearest vitamin store and buy out their supply of iron tablets. As mentioned, an excess of iron may lead to an increase in infection. Since iron deficiency may occur in the absence of anemia, the most reliable way to determine iron status is by performing blood tests: total serum iron, transferrin iron binding capacity, and blood ferritin. The recommended daily dietary allowance for iron in adult males is 15 milligrams and in adult females is 18 milligrams and this includes iron obtained from the diet. Amounts taken in excess, which may be necessary in some individuals to correct anemia, should be monitored and the need for iron should be established before it is taken in supplement form. The best natural sources of iron are liver, kidney, meats, eggs, apricots, brewer's yeast and wheat germ. Cooking acidic foods in iron containers also adds iron to the diet.

ZINC

Zinc deficiency, like iron, can impair a variety of immune responses and defense mechanisms. The mineral deficiency most frequently found in humans is zinc deficiency and since there are no major body storage depots for zinc, a deficiency may easily be produced.[4] Zinc deficiency produces atrophy of the thymus gland, spleen, lymph nodes and intestinal lymphoid tissues resulting in depletion of both T- and B-lymphocyte populations[3,4,5,98] as well as diminished capacity of these lymphocytes to destroy cancerous tumor cells.[4,99] In zinc deficiency antibody production is severely depressed.[4,100,101] The ability of macrophages and granulocytes to entrap and poison invading microbes is impaired in zinc deficiency.[4,102] In contrast, an excess of zinc impairs the ability of these same white blood cells to migrate and engulf microbes.[3,4,103] Generally, zinc has a stimulating effect on all replicating cells, including those involved in the immune response.[4]

Once again, the trick is to obtain enough zinc but avoid an excess. Adults, both males and females, should get about 15 milligrams of zinc per day, but analysis of 'well-rounded' diets served at cafeterias and hospitals show that only 8 to 11 milligrams of zinc per day is provided in the diet.[104] About 30 per cent of dietary zinc is absorbed,[105] so that an oral supplement of 15 milligrams per day may be good insurance against depletion and certainly would be considered safe. However, when men participate in sexual activity they may experience increased zinc excretion. Heavy foreplay and a single orgasm will rid the male body of about one milligram of zinc.[104] Superimposed upon a deficient diet this excretion of zinc alone could lead to impaired immunity.

There are several methods of determining zinc status. This metal can be tested for in the blood, although hair analysis for zinc should also be performed since blood values alone may be spurious.[106] The best dietary sources for zinc are meats, fish and eggs.[40,104] Cereal grains, peanuts and soybeans and their fibers inhibit the absorption of zinc (as well as iron, magnesium and calcium)[107,108,109,110] and a reduction of these foods in the diet may be prudent. Dietary calcium may interfere with zinc absorption.[104] Oral zinc supplements greater than 15 milligrams per day should be monitored because zinc excess interferes with iron absorption and may cause depression of blood copper levels as well as a decreased number of white blood cells.[104]

CALCIUM
When human phagocytes and macrophages react to the presence of foreign invaders they immediately absorb calcium from their microenvironment and without calcium are unable to manufacture the poisonous substances used to kill the invaders.[111,112] The presence of calcium ions also increases the attachment of foreign organisms and bacteria to macrophages and is required for the ingestion process of these organisms.[21] Calcium appears to be required for the production of fever.[20] The first component of the complement system is held together by a calcium-dependent bond[29] and calcium is required for activation of the classic pathway of complement activation.[4,29] The function of cytotoxic T-lymphocytes in antigen-bearing target cell lysis absolutely is calcium dependent.[28] No less than 800 milligrams of calcium should be obtained by adults daily, an amount easily supplied by four ounces of hard cheese, three cups of milk or four cups of cottage cheese. Growing adults between ages 11–18 need 50 per cent more calcium (1,200 milligrams per day).

MAGNESIUM
Magnesium is required for the activation of the alternative pathway of the complement system and for forma-

tion of some of the components.[4,11,29] Magnesium is necessary for the ingestion process employed by phagocytes and macrophages to clear the body of antigenic material.[21] Both hyperplasia and atrophy of the thymus gland can occur in magnesium deficiency with the resulting loss of cell–mediated immunocompetence.[4,113] In experimental animals kept on magnesium deficient diets there is a reduction in antibody levels.[4,114,115] Some types of cancers (malignant lymphoma and myeloid leukemia) appear to increase in experimental animals if they are kept on low magnesium diets, and the longer the deficient diet is maintained, the more these animals become susceptible to these cancers even if they have previously acquired immunity.[113,116,117] The function of cytotoxic T–lymphocytes regarding their interaction with antigen–bearing target cells resulting in the lysis of the target cell has been shown to require the presence of magnesium.[28] In order to properly metabolize calcium and for the competence of the immune system, no less than 350 milligrams of magnesium should be obtained daily for adult males and 300 millgrams for adult females. The best sources of magnesium are nuts and cooked green leafy vegetables. The richest source is sea snails. Most of these foods are difficult to eat in the quantity required so that magnesium tablets might be the easiest way to obtain that amount of magnesium.

IODINE

When phagocytes and granulocytes are actively engaged in the destruction of bacteria, fungi or viruses they produce toxic substances which they combine with iodine.[18,20,21] The iodine is supplied either by removing it from thyroid hormones or from its free state circulating in the blood. Since seaweed is rich in iodine, it is marketed in the form of kelp tablets. One tablet per day supplies the recommended daily allowance of 150 micrograms. Virtually 100 per cent of dietary iodine is absorbed[105] and those who consume commercially produced baked goods, milk and dairy products, convenience and fast foods and Red Dye Number 3 (used as a coloring agent in many processed foods) may have iodine overloads.[118] Excess iodine impairs antibody function and diminishes lymphocyte responses to foreign substances.[119] Iodine levels and thyroid hormones can be determined by blood tests. Natural sources of iodine are ocean fish and sea foods.

COPPER

A deficit or excess of copper produced experimentally has been reported to increase the severity of infections in experimental animals.[4,5,120,121,122] Humans who have inherited diseases involving defects in copper metabolism suffer from low blood copper levels and frequent infections.[123] Fortunately, copper deficiencies in humans are rare and occur only in premature infants and patients who are being fed by intravenous feedings.[104,123] The foods we eat and the water we drink supply the average adult with 3 to 5 milligrams per day.[104] Since the actual adult need is between 2 and 3 milligrams per day,[124] an accumulation of excess copper is likely. Copper plumbing delivery systems supply most of the copper from drinking water and copper sulfate is added to reservoir water to kill the algae (this also works in aquariums although the fish may not survive). Infrequently used faucets accumulate the most copper, especially if the water is 'soft'. 'Hard' water may protect against copper by coating the pipes with lime. Soft-drink dispensers with copper tubing contribute copper as well. The foods with the greatest copper content are liver, oysters, soybeans, wheat germ, cocoa, chocolate and dried yeast. Oral supplements containing copper should be avoided since these will add to the body burden. Copper excess will accentuate a zinc deficiency and may interfere with vitamin B_6.[104] Copper status can be determined by both blood and hair analysis.

SELENIUM

Mild selenium (named after the moon goddess, Selene) excess, as mentioned earlier, seems to be involved synergistically with vitamin E in immune functions.[3,4,5,91] Antibody production depends upon selenium[5,125] and white blood cells cannot produce their bactericidal effects without it.[126] The ingestion activity of macrophages and granulocytes is decreased in selenium deficiency and T-lymphocytes appear to be coated by substances that suppress their response to antigens and proliferation signals.[4] The recommended daily dietary adult allowance for selenium is from 50 to 200 micrograms.[124] The 'average' diet probably contains only 25 to 60 micrograms, so supplements of selenium need to be considered.[127] Selenium becomes toxic when intake is over 1,000 micrograms per day, but oral supplementation of 200 to 400 micrograms should be considered safe. Natural sources of selenium are garlic, liver, brewer's yeast and eggs. There is evidence that where food is obtained and eaten from selenium-adequate soils there is a low cancer rate and the reverse is also true. For instance, the people of Rapid City, South Dakota have the highest blood selenium levels and they have the lowest cancer rates.[127] The people of Lima, Ohio have low blood levels of selenium and a cancer rate twice that of Rapid City. Other selenium-poor states are Connecticut, Illinois, Oregon, Massachusetts, Rhode Island, New York, Delaware and The District of Columbia. Blessed with selenium are North and South Dakota, Colorado, Wyoming, Kansas, Nebraska, Arizona, Utah, Texas, Oklahoma, Louisiana and Alabama. Selenium levels can be determined from hair analysis as well as blood, but hair may be more accurate.[104,106]

Toxic Minerals

Toxic minerals are those which when taken into the body have adverse effects or interfere with normal metabolism. Cadmium, lead, mercury and nickel are toxic metals which wreak subtle havoc on the immune system.[5] Subtoxic quantities of cadmium increase susceptibility to viral infections[128] and inhibit antibody production.[129] Excess mercury and lead accumulation causes immunological changes comparable to those caused by an excess of cadmium.[128] If nickel is added to the media of cultured cells it can suppress the synthesis of interferon.[130] Excess accumulation of chromium and vanadium is toxic to white blood cells.[131] Part of the effect of toxic metals also is found in their interference with the nutritional minerals: zinc, iron, selenium, magnesium and calcium.[104,105]

Where do these toxic minerals come from? Significant amounts of cadmium are found in cigarette smoke, margarine, anchovies, some canned fruits and beverages, wheat, sugar, molasses, alcoholic drinks and 'soft' water (coursing through any kind of plumbing).[104,105] Sources of mercury include large ocean fish (tuna, shark and sword), interior paints (vaporizes from the paint) and laxatives that contain calomel (mercurous chloride).[104,105] Lead will be found in cigarette smoke, tap water (lead plumbing), lead-based paints, lead seams on tin cans (dissolves into contents), automobile exhaust, newsprint, colored inks, vegetables from roadside gardens and bone meal (90 per cent of lead is stored in the skeleton).[104,105] The only significant sources of nickel are in cigarette smoke, margarine and hydrogenated oils.[104,105] Toxic excesses of chromium occur only in chromate industrial workers,[105] but the vanadium contained in the overconsumption of olive, corn or soybean oil, gelatin, black pepper and olives[104] may be significant. Toxic minerals can be tested for in blood, hair and urine. Blood and urine may be appropriate for acute exposures, but hair analysis appears to be the most accurate method of determining chronic exposures.[106] Toxic mineral accumulation can be countered by both avoidance of the source and the proper use of nutritional substances (vitamin C, selenium, zinc, and some amino acids).

Amino Acids

Protein is made by linking one amino acid to another in long chains. High quality protein consumed and digested efficiently will provide amino acids which the body then uses for its own purposes. The importance of protein has already been discussed, but several amino acids deserve special comment.

L-LYSINE

L-Lysine has been used as a successful therapeutic agent in the suppression of herpes virus infections.[132] Another amino acid, L-Arginine, appears to encourage herpes virus infections.[133] Herpes viruses are protected by coats which are rich in L-Arginine and the viruses require L-Arginine for this purpose. Decreasing the amount of L-Arginine or increasing the amount of L-Lysine suppresses the virus. The herpes viruses have been linked to encephalitis and cancer.[132] Cytomegalovirus is a herpes virus that has an extremely high correlation to a rare skin cancer, Kaposi's sarcoma.[134] Since L-Lysine appears to suppress herpes simplex viruses, it may have some use in suppressing cytomegalovirus infections.

There is evidence that macrophages produce an enzyme, arginase, which has the ability to cause a decrease of L-Arginine[16] by converting it to the waste product, urea, and to another amino acid, L-Ornithine. The depletion of L-Arginine may lead to the inhibition of cellular function or cytostasis of cancerous cells.[16] The ingestion of large amounts of L-Arginine or L-Ornithine (which inhibits the action of the enzyme, arginase, resulting in a buildup of L-Arginine[135]) may provide a rich medium for both viral and cancerous cell growth. Avoiding L-Arginine-rich foods such as cereals, grains, nuts, seeds and chocolate and consuming high quality protein foods may aid in producing L-Lysine dominance. L-Lysine tablets can be purchased in health food stores. The suggested maintenance dosage for adults is 500 to 1,000 milligrams per day.[132]

DIMETHYLGLYCINE

The formation of the amino acid, dimethylglycine, occurs in the normal metabolism of the B vitamin, choline,[76] or in the synthesis of the amino acid, glycine, from choline.[136] Dimethylglycine, given orally, has been shown to stimulate a fourfold increase in antibody production in response to antigenic stimulation and to produce a threefold increase in the function of lymphocytes when stimulated with antigens in humans.[137] Since antigens are constantly present, dimethylglycine may be very valuable in producing immunopotentiation on a day to day basis. Remarkably small amounts, 120 milligrams, given over a ten-week period to normal male and female adults produce the effect.[137] Toxicity studies have revealed that there are no toxicological effects in experimental animals from dimethylglycine.[138] Dimethylglycine is available in the pure form in 90 milligram tablets which can be placed under the tongue until they are dissolved.

Healthful Habits

Now that the recipe for manufacturing steel dolls is fairly complete, it becomes apparent that just fabricating steel dolls is not enough. Like other machinery steel dolls need to be cared for. It is necessary that steel dolls avoid becoming rusted by not only consuming optimal nutrients, but by practicing other healthful habits.

Getting adequate rest is essential and it appears that somewhere near seven hours per day is associated with longevity. Less than four hours per day or more than ten hours may shorten life.[139] Physical exercise on a daily or every other day basis is associated with greater health[139] and may be considered a resistance factor. Not only does a daily workout put a glow on your cheeks, it appears to release the chemical, endogenous pyrogen, which causes body temperatures to rise and this in turn increases the efficiency of white blood cells to fight infections and also retards the production of bacteria and viruses.[20,140] Increases in body temperature enhance the activity of white blood cells to fight cancer as well.[141]

Avoiding stress, depression and grief or at least properly dealing with them may also be essential since all of these effects on the psyche have a high association with suppression of the immune system.[142,143,144] The effects of stress, grief and depression appear to be mediated through the effects of corticosteroids and adrenalin produced by the small glands perched on top of each kidney, the adrenal glands.[142] There appears to be a particularly significant effect from depression, grief (over loss of a loved one) and feelings of hopelessness on the immune system with an apparent decrease in the ability to protect the body from cancer.[142,144,145]

Maintaining ideal body weight seems essential since the incidence and severity of infectious diseases is considerably higher in obese people. Deficiencies of zinc and iron are often found in overweight individuals. The incidence of cancers of the breast, prostrate and colon appears to be higher in obese persons.[3,4]

The overconsumption of alcohol not only directly affects the ability of white blood cells to accumulate at the site of an infection,[146] but also causes the loss of nutrients which are vital for optimal immune system functions. At particular risk of deficiency are protein,[147] folic acid,[148] zinc,[104,105] calcium[149] and vitamin E.[150] If alcoholic excess has led to liver disease, then immunosuppression with decreased T-lymphocytes is the rule rather than the exception.[151]

Many drugs are known to suppress the immune response. Especially effective are corticosteroids,[142,145,146,152] antibiotics,[153] tranquilizers[153,154,155] and marijuana.[156,157] Very recent evidence has shown Isobutyl Nitrite to suppress a variety of immune responses.[158] Both Amyl- and Isobutyl Nitrite are known to be capable of causing cancer even after a single dose.[158,159] The popular tonic, ginseng, may even be more potent than corticosteroids in suppressing lymphocyte function.[160]

We live on a planet filled with microorganisms and antigens. Every facet of our existence exposes us to contact with viruses, bacteria, fungi and a multiplicity of other parasitic or potentially parasitic life forms. Considering the continuous nature of our exposure to microorganisms it is surprising that infections are not more common. The best results in improving immunity will be obtained by both reducing the exposure to the risk factors and improving the resistance of humans to environmental threats. The most commonly acquired immunodeficiency is due to malnutrition[161] and optimal nutrition is one way of supporting resistance.

Since humans are individuals and vary greatly in their requirements, utilization and excretion of nutrients[162] — nutrients themselves depend upon each other and are interrelated — it is logical to have oneself evaluated before blindly consuming vitamin, mineral and amino acid supplements. Even general advice about protein, fat and carbohydrates may be inaccurate when applied to some individuals, especially those with liver disorders. Seek the advice of a competent health care professional or nutritionist who can perform blood, urine, hair and physical analyses.

A practical preventive program must consider the individual person and identify and alter those variables which contribute to the body's resistance and susceptibility. Perhaps only in this manner can one bestow upon the glass doll the characteristics of steel which when struck will emit pleasant musical notes.

References

1. Wylie, C. M.: 'The definition and measurement of health and disease.' *Public Health Report*, February, 1970; 85(2):100–04.
2. Cheraskin, E.; Ringsdorf, Jr, W. M. and Clark, J. W.: *Diet and Disease*. New Canaan, Connecticut: Keats Publishing, Inc., 1968.
3. Chandra, R. K.: 'Immunodeficiency in undernutrition and overnutrition.' *Nutrition Reviews*, June, 1981; 39(6):225–31.
4. Levy, J. A.: 'Effects of sex hormones, nutrition and aging on the immune response. II. Nutrition and the immune system.' In: Stites, D. P.; Stobo, J. D.; *et al*. (Eds.): *Basic and Clinical Immunology*, 4th Edition. Los Altos, California: Lange Medical Publications, 1982; pp. 297–305.
5. Chandra, R. K.: 'Nutrition, immunity and infection: present knowledge and future directions.' *The Lancet*, March 26, 1983; I:688–91.
6. Scrimshaw, N. S.; Taylor, C. E. and Gordon, J. E.: In: *Interactions of Nutrition and Infection*, WHO monograph series 57, Geneva, 1968; pp. 60–142.
7. Suskind, R. M.: *Malnutrition and the Immune Response*. New York: Raven Press, 1977.

8. Ammann, A. J. and Fudenberg, H. H.: 'Section III. Clinical Immunology: Immunodeficiency disease.' In: Stites, D. P.; Stobo, J. D.; *et al.* (Eds.): *Basic and Clinical Immunology*, 4th Edition. Los Altos, California: Lange Medical Publications, 1982; pp. 395–429.

9. Solomans, N. W. and Keusch, G. T.: 'Nutritional implications of parasitic infections.' *Nutrition Reviews*, April, 1981; 39(4):149–61.

10. Anonymous. 'Severity of measles in malnutrition.' *Nutrition Reviews*, July, 1982; 40(7):203–5.

11. Hokama, Y. and Nakamura, R. M.: *Immunology and Immunopathology, Basic Concepts*. Boston, Massachusetts: Little, Brown and Company, 1982.

12. Weksler, M. E. and Hausman, P. B.: 'Effects of sex hormones, nutrition and aging on the immune response. III. Effects of aging on the immune response.' In: Stites, D. P.; Stobo, J. D.; *et al.* (Eds.): *Basic and Clinical Immunology*, 4th Edition. Los Altos, California: Lange Medical Publications, 1982; pp. 306–13.

13. Chandra, R. K.; Joshi, P.; *et al.*: 'Nutrition and immunocompetence of the elderly. Effect of short term nutritional supplementation on cell-mediated immunity and lymphocyte subsets.' *Nutrition Research*, 1982; 2:223–32.

14. Katz, D. H.: 'The immune system: an overview.' In: Stites, D. P.; Stobo, J. D.; *et al.* (Eds.): *Basic and Clinical Immunology*, 4th Edition. Los Altos, California: Lange Medical Publications, 1982; pp. 13–20.

15. Schwartz, B. D.: 'The human major histocompatibility HLA complex.' In: Stites, D. P.; Stobo,

J. D.; *et al*. (Eds.): *Basic and Clinical Immunology*, 4th Edition. Los Altos, California: Lange Medical Publications, 1982; pp. 52–64.

16. Werb, Z.: 'Phagocytic cells: chemotaxis and effector functions of macrophages and granulocytes. I. Macrophages.' In: Stites, D. P.; Stobo, J. D.; *et al*. (Eds.): *Basic and Clinical Immunology*, 4th Edition. Los Altos, California: Lange Medical Publications, 1982; pp. 109–18.

17. Goldstein, I. M.: 'Phagocytic cells: chemotaxis and effector functions of macrophages and granulocytes. II. Granulocytes.' In: Stites, D. P.; Stobo, J. D.; *et al*. (Eds.): *Basic and Clinical Immunology*, 4th Edition. Los Altos, California: Lange Medical Publications, 1982; pp. 119–23.

18. Klebanoff, S. J.: 'Oxygen metabolism and the toxic properties of phagocytes.' *Annals of Internal Medicine*, September, 1980; 93(3):480–89.

19. McCord, J. M. and Fridovich, I.: 'The biology and pathology of oxygen radicals.' *Annals of Internal Medicine*, July, 1978; 89(1):122–7.

20. Drutz, D. J. and Mills, J.: 'Immunity and Infection.' In: Stites, D. P.; Stobo, J. D.; *et al*. (Eds.): *Basic and Clinical Immunology*, 4th Edition. Los Altos, California: Lange Medical Publications, 1982; pp. 209–32.

21. Kimura, L. H.: 'Immunity and infections.' In: Hokama, Y. and Nakamura, R. M.: *Immunology and Immunopathology, Basic Concepts*. Boston, Massachusetts: Little, Brown and Company, 1982; pp. 457–91.

22. Benjamini, E.; Rennick, D. M. and Sell, S.: 'Tumor immunology.' In: Stites, D. P.; Stobo,

J. D.; *et al.* (Eds.): *Basic and Clinical Immunology*, 4th Edition. Los Altos, California: Lange Medical Publications, 1982; pp. 233–49.

23. Editorial: 'T-Lymphocytes.' *The Lancet*, April 3, 1982; I:778–9.

24. Reinherz, E. L. and Schlossman, S. F.: 'The differentiation and function of T-Lymphocytes.' *Cell*, April, 1980; 19:821–27.

25. Douglas, S. D.: 'Development and structure of cells in the immune system.' In: Stites, D. P.; Stobo, J. D.; *et al.* (Eds.): *Basic and Clinical Immunology*, 4th Edition. Los Altos, California: Lange Medical Publications, 1982; pp. 65–88.

26. Theofilopoulos, A. N.: 'Autoimmunity.' In: Stites, D. P.; Stobo, J. D.; *et al.* (Eds.): *Basic and Clinical Immunology*, 4th Edition. Los Altos, California: Lange Medical Publications, 1982; pp. 156–88.

27. Alexander, G. J. M.; Nouri-Aria, K-T.; *et al.*: 'Contrasting relations between suppressor-cell function and suppressor-cell number in chronic liver disease.' *The Lancet*, June 11, 1983; I:1291–3.

28. Henney, C. S.: 'Immune mechanisms in tissue damage. II. Cell-mediated cytotoxicity.' In: Stites, D. P.; Stobo, J. D.; *et al.* (Eds.): *Basic and Clinical Immunology*, 4th Edition. Los Altos, California. Lange Medical Publications, 1982; pp. 150–5.

29. Cooper, N. R.: 'The complement system.' In: Stites, D. P.; Stobo, J. D.; *et al.* (Eds.): *Basic and Clinical Immunology*, 4th Edition. Los Altos, California: Lange Medical Publications, 1982; pp. 124–35.

30. Siegel, I. and Gleicher, N.: 'The red army.' *The Sciences*, January/February, 1983; 23(1):30–4.

31. Rocklin, R. E.: 'Mediators of cellular immunity.' In: Stites, D. P.; Stobo, J. D.; *et al*. (Eds.): *Basic and Clinical Immunology*, 4th Edition. Los Altos, California: Lange Medical Publications, 1982; pp. 97–108.

32. Editorial: 'Human interferon as a therapeutic agent — current status.' *The New England Journal of Medicine*, June 23, 1983; 308(25):1530–1.

33. May, J. M.: 'The ecology of human disease.' *Annals of the New York Academy of Sciences*, December 8, 1960; 84(17):789–94.

34. Anderson, K. E.; Conney, A. H. and Kappas, A.: 'Nutritional influences on chemical biotransformations in humans.' *Nutrition Reviews*, June, 1982; 40(6):161–71.

35. Kinlen, L. J.: 'Meat and fat consumption and cancer mortality: a study of strict religious orders in Britain.' *The Lancet*, April 24, 1982; I:946–9.

36. Graham, S.; Dayal, H.; *et al*.: 'Diet in the epidemiology of cancer of the colon and rectum.' *Journal of the National Cancer Institute*, 1978; 61:709–14.

37. Hentges, D. J.: 'Does diet influence human fecal microflora composition?' *Nutrition Reviews*, October, 1980; 38(10):329–36.

38. Mendeloff, A. I.: 'Appraisal of "Diet, Nutrition and Cancer".' *The American Journal of Clinical Nutrition*, March, 1983; 37(3):495–8.

39. Whelan, E. M.: 'Scare talk about foods and cancer.' *Nutrition and the M.D.* August, 1982; VIII(8):1–2.

40. Underwood, E. J.: 'Changes in trace metals in protein or energy restriction.' *Journal of Human Nutrition*, 1978; 32:253–7.

41. Uldall, P. R.; *et al.*: 'Linoleic acid and transplantation.' *The Lancet*, 1975; II:128–9.

42. McHugh, M. I.; *et al.*: 'Immunosuppression with polyunsaturated fatty acids in renal transplantation.' *Transplantation*, 1977; 24:263–7.

43. Parke, D. V. and Ioannides, C.: 'The role of nutrition in toxicology.' In: Darby, W. J.; Broquist, H. P. and Olson, R. E. (Eds.):. *Annual Review of Nutrition*, Palo Alto, California: Annual Reviews, Inc., 1981; I:207–34.

44. Hedgecock, L. W.: 'Effect of dietary fatty acids and protein intake on experimental tuberculosis.' *Journal of Bacteriology*, 1955; 70:415–20.

45. Schole, J.; *et al.*: 'Belastrung, ernahrung, und resistenz.' *Forschr Tierphysiol Tierernaehr* Suppl. 9 Hamburg: Verlag Paul Parey, 1978.

46. Herbert, V.: 'Epidemiology, diet and killer diseases.' *The American Journal of Clinical Nutrition*, April, 1982; 34(4):592–3.

47. Fiser, Jr., R. J.; *et al.*: 'Altered immune functions in hypercholesterolemic monkeys.' *Infection and Immunity*, 1973; 8:105–9.

48. Klurfeld, D. M.; *et al.*: 'Alteration of host defenses paralleling cholesterol-induced atherogenesis. II. Immunologic studies of rabbits.' *Journal of Medicine*, 1979; 10:49–64.

49. Chen, S. S-H.: 'Requirement of cholesterol for successful blastogenesis in mitogen-stimulated lymphocytes.' *Federation Proceedings*, 1978; 37:377.

50. Mayes, P. A.: 'Metabolism of lipids.' In: Harper, H. A.; *et al.*: *Review of Physiological Chemistry*. Los Altos, California: Lange Medical Publications, 1977; pp. 280–320.

51. Matthews-Roth, M. M.: 'Neutropenia and beta-carotene.' *The Lancet*, July 24, 1982; II:222.
52. Schoenfeld, Y.; *et al.*: 'Neutropenia induced by hypercarotenaemia.' *The Lancet*, May 29, 1982; I:1245.
53. Kominos, S. D.; *et al.*: 'Introduction of *Pseudomonus aeruginosa* into a hospital via vegetables.' *Applied Microbiology*, 1972; 24:567–70.
54. Schimpff, S. C.: 'Surveillance cultures.' *The Journal of Infectious Diseases*, 1981; 144:81–4.
55. Remington, J. S. and Schimpff, S. C.: 'Please don't eat the salads.' *The New England Journal of Medicine*, 1981; 304:433–4.
56. Axelrod, A. E. and Trakatellis, A. C.: 'Relationship of pyridoxine to immunological phenomena.' *Vitamins and Hormones*, 1964; 22:591–607.
57. Stoerk, H. C. and Zucker, T. F.: 'Nutritional effects on the development and atrophy of the thymus.' *Proceedings of the Society for Experimental Biology and Medicine*, 1944; 56:151–3.
58. Hodges, R. E.; *et al.*: 'Factors affecting human antibody response. IV. Pyridoxine deficiency.' *The American Journal of Clinical Nutrition*, 1962; 11:180–6.
59. Hodges, R. E.; *et al.*: 'Factors affecting human antibody response. V. Combined deficiencies of pantothenic acid and pyridoxine.' *The American Journal of Clinical Nutrition*, 1962; 11:187–99.
60. Lederer, W. H.; Kumar, M. and Axelrod, A. E.: 'Effects of pantothenic acid deficiency on cellular antibody synthesis in rats.' *The Journal of Nutrition*, 1975; 105:17–25.
61. Gross, R. L. and Newberne, P. M.: 'Role of nutri-

90 / *How To Fortify* . . .

tion in immunologic function.' *Physiological Reviews*, 1980; 60:188–302.

62. Gross, R. L.; *et al.*: 'Depressed cell-mediated immunity in megaloblastic anemia due to folic acid deficiency.' *The American Journal of Clinical Nutrition*, 1975; 28:225–32.

63. MacCuish, A. C.; *et al.*: 'PHA responsiveness and subpopulations of circulating lymphocytes in pernicious anemia.' *Blood*, 1974; 44:849–55.

64. Robertson, J. S.; Hsia, Y. E. and Scully, K. J.: 'Defective leucocyte metabolism in human cobalamin deficiency: impaired propionate oxidation and serine biosynthesis reversible by cyanocobalamin therapy.' *Journal of Laboratory and Clinical Medicine*, 1976; 87:89–97.

65. Axelrod, A. E.; *et al.*: 'Circulating antibodies in vitamin-deficiency states: I. Pyridoxine, riboflavin and pantothetic acid deficiencies.' *Proceedings of the Society for Experimental Biology and Medicine*, 1947; 66:137–40.

66. Prinz, W.; *et al.*: 'The effect of ascorbic acid supplementation on some parametyers of the human immunological defence system.' *International Journal for Vitamin and Nutrition Research*, 1977; 47:248–57.

67. Murphy, B. L.; *et al.*: 'Ascorbic acid (vitamin C) and its effects on parainfluenza type III virus infection in cotton-topped marmosets.' *Laboratory Animal Science*, 1974; 24:229–32.

68. Fraser, R. C.; *et al.*, 'The effect of variations in vitamin C intake on the cellular immune response of guinea pigs.' *The American Journal of Clinical Nutrition*, 1978; 33:839–47.

69. Stankova, L.; *et al.*: 'Ascorbate and phagocyte function.' *Infection and Immunity*, 1975; 12:252–6.

70. Sandler, J. A.; Gallin, J. I. and Vaughan, M.: 'Effects of serotonin, carbamylcholine, and ascorbic acid on leucocyte cyclic GMP and chemotaxis.' *Journal of Cell Biology*, 1975; 67:480–4.

71. Siegel, B. V.: 'Enhancement of interferon production by poly(rI)poly(rC) in mouse cell cultures by ascorbic acid.' *Nature*, 1975; 254:431–2.

72. Dahl, H. and Degre, M.: 'The effect of ascorbic acid on production of human interferon and the antiviral activity in vitro.' *Acta Pathologica et Microbiologica Scandinavica, Section B: Microbiology*, 1976; 84B:280–4.

73. Geber, W. F.; Lefkowitz, S. S. and Hung, C. Y.: 'Effect of ascorbic acid, sodium salicylate and caffeine on the serum interferon level in response to viral infection.' *Pharmacology*, 1975; 13:228–33.

74. Dieter, M. P.: 'Further studies on the relationship between vitamin C and thymic humoral factor.' *Proceedings of the Society for Experimental Biology and Medicine*, 1971; 136:316–22.

75. Green, L. C. and Tannenbaum, S. R.: 'Nitrate and Nitrite in food.' *Nutrition and the M.D.*, May, 1982; VIII(5):1–3.

76. Harper, H. A.: 'The water soluble vitamins.' In: Harper, H. A.; *et al.*: *Review of Physiological Chemistry*. Los Altos, California: Lange Medical Publications, 1977; pp 156–81.

77. Klenner, F. R.: 'Significance of high daily intake of ascorbic acid in preventive medicine.' In: Williams, R. J. and Kalita, D. K. (Eds.): *A Physician's Hand-*

book on *Orthomolecular Medicine*. New York: Pergamon Press, 1977; pp 51–9.

78. Nauss, K. M.; Mark, D. A. and Suskind, R. M.: 'The effect of vitamin A deficiency on the in vitro cellular immune response of rats.' *The Journal of Nutrition*, 1979; 109:1815–23.

79. Bang, B. G.; Bang, F. B. and Foard, M. A.: 'Lymphocyte depression induced in chickens on diets deficient in vitamin A and other components.' *The American Journal of Pathology*, 1972; 68:147–62.

80. Mohanram, M.; Reddy, V. and Mishra, S.: 'Lysozyme activity in plasma and leucocytes in malnourished children.' *The British Journal of Nutrition*, 1974; 32:313–16.

81. Cohen, B. E.; *et al.*: 'Reversal of postoperative immunosuppression in man by vitamin A.' *Surgery, Gynecology and Obstetrics*, 1979; 149:658–62.

82. Cohen, B. E. and Elin, R. J.; 'Vitamin A-induced nonspecific resistance to infection.' *The Journal of Infectious Diseases*, 1974; 129:597–600.

83. Farris, W. A. and Erdman, J. W.: 'Protracted hypervitaminosis A following long-term, low-level intake.' *The Journal of the American Medical Association*, March 5, 1982; 247(9):1317–8.

84. Herbert, V.: 'Toxicity of 25,000 I.U. vitamin A supplements in "health" food users.' *The American Journal of Clinical Nutrition*, July, 1982; 36(1):185–6.

85. Stampfer, M. J.; Willett, W. and Hennekens, C. H.: 'Carotene, carrots, and white blood cells.' *The Lancet*, September 11, 1982; II:615.

86. Tengerdy, R. P.; Heinzerling, R. H. and Mathias,

M. M.: 'Effect of vitamin E on disease resistance and immune responses.' In: de Dune, C. and Hayaishi, O. (Eds.): *Tocopherol, Oxygen and Biomembranes*. Amsterdam: Elsevier/North-Holland Biomedical Press, 1978; pp 191–200.

87. Ayres, Jr., S. and Mihan, R.: 'Is vitamin E involved in the autoimmune mechanism?' *Cutis*, 1978; 21:321–5.

88. Ellis, R. P. and Vorhies, M. W.: 'Effect of supplementary dietary vitamin E on the serologic response of swine to an Escherichia coli bacterin.' *Journal of the American Veterinary Medical Association*, 1976; 168:231–2.

89. Nockels, C. F.: 'Protective effects of supplemental vitamin E against infection.' *Federation Proceedings*, 1979; 38:2134–8.

90. Corwin, L. M. and Shloss, J.: 'Influence of vitamin E on the mitogenic response of murine lymphoid cells.' *The Journal of Nutrition*, 1980; 110:916–23.

91. Heinzerling, R. H.; *et al.*: 'Protection of chicks against E. coli infection by dietary supplementation with vitamin E.' *Proceedings of the Society for Experimental Biology and Medicine*, 1974; 146:279–83.

92. Burton, G. W.; Joyce, A. and Ingold, K. U.: 'First proof that vitamin E is major lipid-soluble, chain-breaking antioxidant in human blood plasma.' *The Lancet*, August 7, 1982; II:327.

93. Weinberg, E. D.: 'Nutritional Immunity. Host's attempt to withhold iron from microbial invaders.' *The Journal of the American Medical Association*, 1975; 231:39–41.

94. McFarlane, H.; *et al.*: 'Immunity, transferrin, and

survival in kwashiorkor.' *British Medical Journal*, 1970; 4:268–70.

95. Fletcher, J.; *et al.*: 'Mouth lesions in iron-deficient anemia: relationship to *Candida albicans* in saliva and to impairment of lymphocyte transformation.' *The Journal of Infectious Diseases*, 1975; 131:44–50.

96. Bhaskaram, C. and Reddy, V.: 'Cell-mediated immunity in iron- and vitamin-deficient children.' *British Medical Journal*, 1975; 3:522.

97. Chandra, R. K. and Saraya, A. K.: 'Impaired immunocompetence associated with iron deficiency.' *Journal of Pediatrics*, 1975; 86:899–902.

98. Tanaka, T.; *et al.*: 'Effect of zinc deficiency on lymphoid tissues and on immune functions of A/Jax mice.' *Federation Proceedings*, 1978; 37:931.

99. Fernandes, G.; *et al.*: 'Impairment of cell-mediated immunity functions by dietary zinc deficiency in mice.' *Proceedings of the National Academy of Sciences, USA*, 1979; 76:457–61.

100. Brummerstedt, E.; *et al.*: 'Animal model of human disease. Acrodermatitis enteropathica, zinc malabsorption.' *The American Journal of Pathology*, 1977; 87:725–8.

101. Cunningham-Rundles, C.; *et al.*: 'Increased T lymphocyte function and thymopoietin following zinc repletion in man.' *Federation Proceedings*, 1979; 38:1222.

102. Anonymous. 'Zinc and polymorphonuclear leucocyte function.' *Nutrition Reviews*, October, 1977; 35(10):266–8.

103. Zukoski, C. F.; *et al.*: 'Functional immobilization of peritoneal macrophages by zinc.' *Journal of the Reticuloendothelial Society*, 1974; 16:6a.

104. Pfeiffer, C. C.: *Zinc and Other Micro-Nutrients*. New Canaan, Connecticut: Keats Publishing, Inc., 1978.

105. Schroeder, H. A.: *The Trace Elements and Man*. Old Greenwich, Connecticut: The Devin-Adair Company, 1973.

106. Laker, M.: 'On determining trace element levels in man: The uses of blood and hair.' *The Lancet*, July 31, 1982; II:260–2.

107. Bordin, S. W. and Bordin, G. M.: 'Bran: Roughage that's rough on iron.' *The New England Journal of Medicine*, January 1, 1976; 294(1):57.

108. Oberleas, D. and Prasad, A. S.: 'Factors affecting zinc homeostasis.' In: Prasad, A. S. and Oberleas, D. (Eds.): *Trace Elements in Human Health and Disease*. New York: Academic Press, 1976; pp. 155–62.

109. Reinhold, J. G.; *et al*.: 'Binding of zinc to fiber and other solids of wholemeal bread.' In: Prasad, A. S. and Oberleas, D. (Eds.): *Trace Elements in Human Health and Disease*. New York: Academic Press, 1976; pp 163–80.

110. Fernandez, R. and Phillips, S. F.: 'Components of fiberbind iron in vitro.' *The American Journal of Clinical Nutrition*, January, 1982; 35(1):100–06.

111. Korchak, H. M. and Smolen, J. E.: 'The role of calcium movements in human neutrophil (PMN) activation.' *Federation Proceedings*, 1980; 40:753.

112. Hui, D. Y.; Berebitsky, G. L. and Harmony, J. A. K.: 'Mitogen-stimulated calcium ion accumulation by lymphocytes. Influence of plasma lipoproteins.' *The Journal of Biological Chemistry*, 1979; 254:4666–73.

113. Hass, G. M.; *et al.*: 'Lymphoproliferative and immunologic aspects of magnesium deficiency.' In: Cantin, M. and Seelig, M. (Eds.): *Magnesium in Health and Disease*. Jamaica, New York: Spectrum, 1980; pp 185–200.
114. Alcock, N. W. and Shils, M. E.: 'Serum immuno-globulin G in the magnesium-depleted rat.' *Proceedings of the Society for Experimental Biology and Medicine*, 1974; 145:855–8.
115. Elin, R. J.: 'The effect of magnesium deficiency in mice on serum immunoglobulin concentrations and antibody plaque-forming cells.' *Proceedings of the Society for Experimental Biology and Medicine*, 1975; 148:620–4.
116. Hass, G. M.; *et al.*: 'Magnesium deprivation in the rat causes loss of induced immunity to malignant lymphoma.' *Clinical Research*, 1978; 26:710A.
117. McCreary, P.; Laing, G. and Hass, G.: 'Susceptibility of normal and magnesium-deficient rats to weekly subtumorigenic doses of liver lymphoma cells.' *The American Journal of Pathology*, 1973; 70:89a–90a.
118. Monagan, D.: 'The iodine scare.' *American Health*, September/October, 1982; 1(iv):26.
119. Haggard, D. L.; *et al.*: 'Immunologic effects of experimental iodine toxicosis in young cattle.' *American Journal of Veterinary Research*, 1980; 41:539–43.
120. Newberne, P. M.; Hunt, C. E. and Young, V. R.: 'The role of diet and the reticuloendothelial system in the response of rats to *Salmonella typhimurium* infection.' *The British Journal of Experimental Pathology*, 1968; 49:448–57.

121. Hill, C. H.: 'Influence of time of exposure to high levels of minerals on the susceptibility of chicks to *Salmonella gallinarum.*' *The Journal of Nutrition*, 1980; 110:433–6.

122. Vaughn, V. J. and Weinberg, E. D.: 'Candida albicans dimorphism and virulence: role of copper.' *Mycopathologia*, 1978: 64:39–42.

123. Anonymous. 'Copper intake and immune responses.' *Nutrition Reviews*, April, 1982; 40(4):107–8.

124. Harper, A. E.: 'Recommended dietary allowances — 1980.' *Nutrition Reviews* August, 1980; 30(8):290–4.

125. Spallholz, J. E.; *et al.*: 'Enhanced immunoglobulin M and immunoglobulin G antibody titers in mice fed selenium.' *Infection and Immunity*, 1973; 8:841–2.

126. Boyne, R. and Arthur, J. R.: 'Alterations of neutrophil function in selenium-deficient cattle.' *Journal of Comparative Pathology*, 1979; 89:151–8.

127. Passwater, R. A.: *Cancer and Its Nutritional Therapies*. New Canaan, Connecticut: Keats Publishing, Inc., 1978.

128. Gainer, J. H.: 'Effect of heavy metals and of deficiency of zinc on mortality rates in mice infected with encephalomyocarditis virus.' *American Journal of Veterinary Research*, 1977; 38:869–72.

129. Koller, L. D.; Exon, J. H. and Roan, J. G.: 'Antibody suppression by cadmium.' *Archives of Environmental Health*, 1975; 30:598–601.

130. Treagan, L.: 'Metals and the immune response. A review.' *Research Communications in Chemical Pathology and Pharmacology*, 1975; 12:198–220.

131. Waters, M. D.; *et al.*: 'Metal toxicity for rabbit alveolar macrophages *in vitro.*' *Environmental Research*, 1975; 9:32–47.

132. Griffith, R. S.; Norins, A. L. and Kagan, C.: 'A multicentered study of lysine therapy in herpes simplex infection.' *Dermatologica*, 1978; 156: 257–67.

133. Tankersley, Jr., R. W.: 'Amino acid requirements of herpes simplex virus in human cells.' *Journal of Bacteriology*, 1964; 87:609–13.

134. Drew, W. L.; *et al.*: 'Cytomegalovirus and Kaposi's sarcoma in young homosexual men.' *The Lancet*, July 17, 1982; II:125–7.

135. Rodwell, V. W.: 'Catabolism of amino acids.' In: Harper, H. A.; *et al.*: *Review of Physiological Chemistry*. Los Altos, California: Lange Medical Publications, 1977; pp 337–68.

136. Rodwell, V. W.: 'Biosynthesis of amino acids.' In: Harper, H. A.; *et al.*: *Review of Physiological Chemistry*. Los Altos, California: Lange Medical Publications, 1977; pp 369–390.

137. Graber, C. D.; *et al.*: 'Immunomodulating properties of dimethylglycine in humans.' *The Journal of Infectious Diseases*, January, 1981; 143(1):101–5.

138. Meduski, J. W.: 'Nutritional evaluation of the results of the 157-day subchronical estimation of N,N-dimethylglycine toxicity carried out in the Nutritional Research Laboratory, University of Southern California School of Medicine.' Pacific Coast Biochemical Conference. July 7–9, 1980; University of California, San Diego.

139. Hammond, E. C.: 'Some preliminary findings on physical complaints from a prospective study of

1,064,004 men and women.' *American Journal of Public Health*, January, 1964; 54(1):11–23.

140. Anonymous. 'Fight infections with exercise.' *Science 82*, July/August, 1982; 3(6):6.

141. Zanker, K. S. and Lange, J.: 'Whole body hyperthermia and natural killer cell activity.' *The Lancet*, May 8, 1982; I:1079–80.

142. Soloman, G. F. and Amkraut, A. A.: 'Psychoneuroendocrinological effects on the immune response.' *Annual Review of Microbiology* Palo Alto, California: Annual Reviews, Inc., 1981; 35:155–84.

143. Jemmott, III, J. D.; *et al.*: 'Academic stress, power motivation, and decrease in secretion rate of salivary secretory immunoglobulin A.' *The Lancet*, June 25, 1983; I:1400–2.

144. Visintainer, M. and Seligman, M.: 'The hope factor.' *American Health*, July/August, 1983; 2(4):58–61.

145. Macek, C.: 'Of mind and morbidity: Can stress and grief depress immunity?' *The Journal of the American Medical Association*, July 23/30, 1982; 248(4):405–7.

146. Editorial: 'Defects of neutrophil function.' *The New England Journal of Medicine*, August 12, 1982; 307(7):434–6.

147. Harper, H. A.: 'The blood, lymph, and cerebrospinal fluid.' In: Harper, H. A.; *et al.*: *Review of Physiological Chemistry*. Los Altos, California: Lange Medical Publications, 1977; pp 559–86.

148. Cherrick, G. R.; *et al.*: 'Observations on hepatic avidity for folate in Laennec's cirrhosis.' *Journal of Laboratory and Clinical Medicine*, 1965; 66:446.

149. Avioli, L. V. and Haddad, J. G.: 'Vitamin D: current concepts.' *Metabolism* 1973; 22:507.

150. Klatskin, G. and Krehl, W. A.: 'The significance of the plasma tocopherol concentration and of tocopherol tolerance tests in liver disease.' *The Journal of Clinical Investigation*, 1950; 29:1528.

151. Anonymous. Malnutrition and anergy in liver disorders.' *Nutrition Reviews*, April, 1982; 40(4):105–6.

152. Webb, Jr., D. R. and Winkelstein, A.: 'Immunosuppression, immunopotentiation, and anti-inflammatory drugs.' In: Stites, D. P.; Stobo, J. D.; *et al*. (Eds.): *Basic and Clinical Immunology*. Los Altos, California: Lange Medical Publications, 1982; pp. 277–92.

153. Huff, B. B. (Ed.): *Physician's Desk Reference*. Oradell, New Jersey: Medical Economics Company, Inc., 1982.

154. Albertini, R. S. and Penders, T. M.: 'Agranulocytosis associated with tricyclics.' *The Journal of Clinical Psychiatry*, 1978; 39:483–5.

155. Ream, R. S. and Kerr, R. O.: 'Neutropenia associated with Maprotiline.' *The Journal of the American Medical Association*, August 20, 1982; 248(7):871.

156. Council on Scientific Affairs: 'Marijuana. Its health hazards and therapeutic potentials.' *The Journal of the American Medical Association*, October 16, 1982; 246(16):1823–7.

157. Nahas, G. G.; Manger, W. M. and Frick, H. C.: 'Marijuana and health.' *The New England Journal of Medicine*, July 22, 1982; 307(4):248.

158. Macek, C.: 'Acquired immunodeficiency syndrome cause(s) still elusive.' *The Journal of the*

American Medical Association, September 24, 1982; 248(12):1423–31.

159. Jorgensen, K. A. and Lawesson, S.: 'Amyl Nitrite and Kaposi's sarcoma in homosexual men.' *The New England Journal of Medicine*, September 30, 1982; 307(14):893–4.

160. Chong, S. K. F.; *et al.*: 'Effect of ginseng saponins and hydrocortisone on phytohaemagglutinin transformation of lymphocytes.' *The Lancet*, September 18, 1982; II:663–4.

161. Sabrado, J.; *et al.*: 'Effect of dietary protein depletion on nonspecific immune responses and survival in the guinea pig.' *The American Journal of Clinical Nutrition*, May, 1983; 37(5):795–801.

162. Williams, R. J.: *Biochemical Individuality*. Austin, Texas: University of Texas Press, 1956.